Raven Press Series in Physiology

Cardiovascular Physiology

Raven Press Series in Physiology
William F. Ganong, M.D., SERIES EDITOR

Cardiovascular Physiology (1988)
Jon Goerke and Allan H. Mines

Membrane Transport and Bioelectricity:
An Introduction to Cellular Physiology (1988)
John H. Byrne and Stanley G. Schultz

Basic Medical Endocrinology (1988)
H. Maurice Goodman

Respiratory Physiology, Second Edition (1986)
Allan H. Mines

Cardiovascular Physiology

Jon Goerke, M.D.   **Allan H. Mines, Ph.D.**

Department of Physiology
University of California School of Medicine
San Francisco, California

Raven Press   New York

Raven Press, 1185 Avenue of the Americas, New York, New York 10036

Made in the United States of America

Library of Congress Cataloging-in-Publication Data

Goerke, Jon.
  Cardiovascular physiology.

  (Raven Press series in physiology)
  Includes bibliographies and index.
  1. Cardiovascular system—Physiology. I. Mines,
Allan H. II. Title. III. Series. [DNLM:
1. Cardiovascular System—physiology. WG 102 G597c]
QP102.G64 1988   612'.1   86-42893
ISBN 0-88167-413-3
ISBN 0-88167-387-0 (soft)

The material contained in this volume was submitted as previously unpublished material, except in the instances in which credit has been given to the source from which some of the illustrative material was derived.

Great care has been taken to maintain the accuracy of the information contained in the volume. However, neither Raven Press nor the editors can be held responsible for errors or for any consequences arising from the use of the information contained herein.

9 8 7 6 5 4 3 2 1

To Betty and Susan

Preface

This text is designed to be used by students involved in a course of organ system physiology at the medical level. The "big picture" is therefore stressed in the attempt to achieve clarity. The book is not intended as a reference text for research scientists. We apologize in advance to them for having given short shrift to the myriad of interesting (but often confounding) secondary and tertiary issues.

This book, like the monograph on Respiratory Physiology published by Raven Press, began as a syllabus first written for our medical and pharmacy students here at UCSF in 1978. It has been updated and rewritten each year since, largely in response to feedback from our students. Those approaches which worked well to further conceptual understanding have been retained. The others have either been dropped or they have been rewritten until they did work well. We are indebted to our medical and pharmacy students for their help in the evolution of this test.

Like the respiration text, this one includes problems to be worked at the end of each chapter, together with answers to those problems. These answers include suggestions as to the logical processes which might have been used in solving the problems. We both believe that the ability to solve problems using physiological information is invaluable to a student in the health sciences. Having been through a course in organ system physiology without having learned to use the information, concepts, normal values, equations, etc., to solve physiological and clinical problems is not terribly useful. Only half the task has been completed. It is not unlike having learned all the rules of the road from a book without having gained the psychomotor skills necessary to drive a car.

As another aid in learning how to use physiology in a problem-solving situation, we have included a chapter in this text which consists of patient cases. These have been very well received by our students. The patient data unfold from the chief complaint, through the present illness, past history, physical exam, laboratory results, cardiac catheterization results, echocardiography, etc. To help the students interpret the clinical information, each clinical finding, each sign and symptom, each laboratory result, etc., is followed by a number in parentheses. Looking up this number at the end of the patient case leads to an explanation of what that particular clinical datum means in physiological terms. There are also questions and calculations followed by numbers in parentheses. The student is meant to do his/her best to answer the question or do the calculation, and then to compare results with the answers at the end of the patient case.

This book will be of interest as a course textbook to medical students, allied health students, and graduate academic students in physiology and related subjects.

Jon Goerke, M.D.
Allan H. Mines, Ph.D.

Contents

Raven Press Series in Physiology

Cardiovascular Physiology

TABLE 1. *Symbols in Cardiovascular Physiology*

Symbol	Definition	Symbol	Definition
A	Alveolar	P_{TM}	Transmural pressure
a	Arterial	PA	Pulmonary artery
Ao	Aorta	PV	Pulmonary vein
AV	Atrioventricular	$\dot{Q}$	Flow (Quantity/Time)
BR	Baroreceptor	$\dot{Q}_T$	Total flow (Quantity/Time)
C	Concentration	r	Radius
dias	Diastolic	R	Resistance
dl	Amount of marker	R_S	Systemic resistance
dt	Time interval	Rv	Venous resistance
E	Equilibrium	RA	Right atrium
EDV	End diastolic volume	RV	Right ventricle
ESV	End systolic volume	S	Stress
E_M	Membrane equilibrium	S_W	Wall stress
F	Force	SA	Sinoatrial
g	Conductance	STPD	Standard temperature, pressure, dry (0°C, 760 mm Hg)
g	Acceleration due to gravity	SV	Stroke volume
h	Height	*t*	Time
h	Wall thickness	v	Venous
HR	Heart rate	V	Volume
I_0	Amount injected	V_{max}	Maximum velocity
k	Slope	η	Fluid viscosity
L	Length	ρ	Specific gravity
LA	Left atrium	.	Time derivative
LV	Left ventricle	-	Mean value
P	Partial pressure		
P	Permeability		
P_{MC}	Mean circulatory pressure		

Thus, PA_{O_2} = Partial pressure of O_2 in alveolar gas
Pa_{O_2} = Partial pressure of O_2 in arterial blood
$\bar{Pa}$ = Mean arterial pressure
$C_{PV}O_2$ = Concentration of O_2 in pulmonary veins

1

Overview of the Circulation

MAIN PURPOSES OF THE CIRCULATION

Perfusion of the central nervous system with oxygenated blood is the main job of the circulation. The terms ''perfusion'' and ''oxygenation'' mean that a pump and an oxygenator are both necessary, and therefore that blood flow through the coronary and pulmonary arteries will have almost equally high priority. The body is quite despotic in enforcing these priorities, and will readily sacrifice a pair of kidneys when the brain is threatened by a severe stress such as a large blood loss.

HOW THE BASIC CIRCUIT WORKS

A Quick Anatomical Look

Before we investigate cardiovascular functions, let's follow blood around the circuit to familiarize ourselves with landmarks as in Fig. 1.1. Starting in the right ventricle, blood is ejected via the pulmonic valve into the pulmonary artery. From here it goes through the small pulmonary arterioles, capillaries, and venules of the lung vascular bed, leaving by way of the pulmonary veins. It then enters the left atrium and goes through the mitral (bicuspid) valve into

1

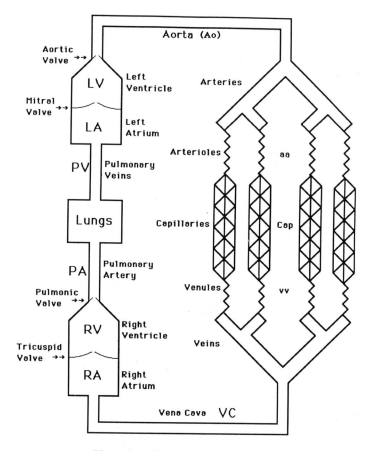

Fig. 1.1. Main parts of circulation.

the left ventricle during its diastolic (relaxing) phase. Blood is ejected from the left ventricle through the aortic valve during systole (ventricular contraction), and passes successively through the aorta, smaller arteries, arterioles, capillaries, venules, veins, and vena cavas to be delivered to the right atrium. Then, passing through the tricuspid valve, it returns to the right ventricle. The average red blood cell takes about a minute to make this circuit.

A More Detailed Look

Figure 1.2 provides more detail about the same blood circuit. Starting again in the right ventricle, pressure increases during ventricular contraction (systole, lasting approximately one-third of the cardiac cycle) and decreases during ventricular relaxation (diastole, lasting approximately two-thirds of the cardiac cycle). This is associated with a pulsatile flow through the pulmonic valve and pulsatile pressures in the pulmonary artery. The pressure drops as the blood traverses the pulmonary arterioles and enters the pulmonary capillary bed. Here the blood comes essentially into an equilibrium with alveolar air where the partial pressure of oxygen (P_{O_2}) is about 100 mm Hg, and the partial pressure of carbon dioxide (P_{CO_2}) is about 40 mm Hg. Since the alveolar air is at atmospheric pressure at end expiration, the partial pressures of the gases dissolved in pulmonary capillary blood must sum to atmospheric pressure. This means taking into account the water vapor (P_{H_2O} = 47 mm Hg) and nitrogen (P_{N_2} = 573 mm Hg) present. A more detailed picture of the gas relationships comes with study of respiratory physiology.

Oxygenated blood, carrying roughly 200 ml of O_2 per liter at a P_{O_2} of 100 mm Hg is thus delivered via the pulmonary veins into the left side of the atrioventricular pumping system. Here again, ventricular systole and diastole produce a pulsatile flow into an arterial system with resulting systolic and diastolic arterial pressures. The flow leaves the aorta through parallel arterial paths to the separate organs. Each of these parallel tissues or organs is therefore exposed to a common driving pressure, equivalent to mean arterial pressure minus mean venous pressure. Blood is thus equally available to all organs, with individual flows being controlled by the arteriolar resistance of each organ.

Once into the tissue capillary beds, the blood unloads **some** (only about 25%) of its oxygen load and takes up an **additional** burden of carbon dioxide. The P_{O_2} averages 40 mm Hg in the venules leaving the tissues, although this varies widely from organ to organ. P_{CO_2} of blood leaving the tissues averages 46 mm Hg.

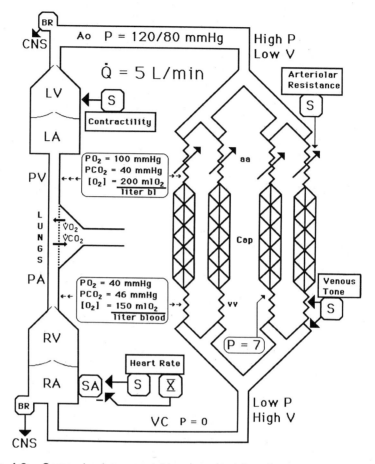

Fig. 1.2. Some circulatory variables. aa, arterioles; Ao, aorta; BR, baroreceptors; Cap, capillaries; CNS, central nervous system; LA, left atrium; LV, left ventricle; P, pressure (Po_2, partial pressure of oxygen; Pco_2, partial pressure of carbon dioxide); PA, pulmonary artery; PV, pulmonary veins; $\dot{Q}$, flow (quantity per time); RA, right atrium; RV, right ventricle; S, sympathetic nervous system; SA, sinoatrial node; V, volume; VC, vena cava; vv, venules; $\underline{X}$, tenth cranial nerve.

Metabolites other than CO_2 are also picked up by the capillary blood and carried away, and substrates such as glucose and fatty acids are delivered to the tissues along with the O_2. Pressure in the huge venous–venular reservoir is quite steady in the supine subject, and serves to drive blood forward through the small resistance of the venous system into the right atrium.

Basic Circulatory Features

Certain features of the circulatory structures need to be understood right from the start.

Arteries versus Veins

The aorta and large arteries are high-pressure, low-volume vessels which serve as an energy reservoir to accept and store a small amount of blood ejected under high pressure during ventricular systole. While the heart is relaxing in diastole, it is disconnected from the aorta, and this relatively small arterial pressure reservoir keeps feeding blood to the periphery. The venules and veins on the other hand are low-pressure, high-volume structures acting as a volume reservoir to feed the ventricular pumps as needed.

Arterioles

As mentioned above, each organ's blood supply is normally determined by its arteriolar resistance. If all these arteriolar faucets were fully opened at one time, however, arterial pressure would rapidly fall, and the brain and heart would not get their special quotas of blood. When arterial blood pressure starts to fall for any reason, the body acts rather despotically and effects a compromise which is more expedient than it is democratic. When possible, the privileged pair, heart and brain, are allowed as much blood as they want by letting them control their own arterioles and by supplying **central** controls to the resistance vessels of the rest of the circulation. The net effect is to maintain arterial blood pressure constant in the face of varying needs and varying supply. Thus, when the supply is short, as it may be following a hemorrhage, blood flow to the skin, extremities, and even the kidneys may be nearly shut off. This can lead to such dire long-term consequences as renal failure, but the rest of the body will have been given at least a temporary lease on life.

Sympathetics and Baroreceptors

The body uses efferent (motor) nerves in the sympathetic nervous system (S in Fig. 1.2) to control arteriolar resistances outside of the brain, heart, and lungs. To supply information for this control system, arterial pressure is continually monitored by arterial baroreceptors (pressure receptors, BR in Fig. 1.2) situated in the carotid sinuses at the bifurcations of the common carotids and in the arch of the aorta. An increase in pressure produces an increase in impulses in the afferent (sensory) nerves serving these structures. High pressure in the carotid sinus sends signals up the glossopharyngeal (ninth cranial) nerves to the brain, and high pressure in the aortic arch increases afferent traffic in sensory fibers contained within the vagus nerve.

The Medulla

These afferent signals are integrated within brain centers lying in the medulla. The result is that when arterial pressure is too high, the medullary centers send fewer efferent impulses via the sympathetics to the arterioles, and these structures relax a bit, allowing some of the aortic pressure to "bleed off." Conversely, a dip in arterial pressure will cause the baroreceptors to send fewer impulses to the medullary cardiovascular centers, resulting in more sympathetic efferent impulses and therefore in increased arteriolar constriction.

Heart Rate, Contractility, and Venous Tone

Along with these signals to manage arteriolar activity, controls are also being applied to the heart and to the venous reservoir. When there is a need to increase the arterial blood pressure, sympathetic impulses cause the heart to beat more rapidly and to put out more blood with each beat (the latter being related to an increase in contractility). At the same time similar signals cause muscles within the walls of the venular reservoir to increase their tone, shrinking the size of the reservoir, increasing reservoir pressure, and thus delivering more blood to the waiting pump.

Efferent Vagal Impulses

A separate control system, involving motor components of the vagus (tenth cranial) nerve ($\overline{X}$ in Fig. 1.2), also participates in these adjustments to blood pressure changes. Even at normal blood pressures there is efferent traffic down the vagus to the sinoatrial (SA) node in the heart. This slows pacemaker activity in this site and thus functions as a continual brake on heart rate.

Integrated Responses

The typical response of the arterial baroreceptor system to high arterial pressure is thus to inhibit sympathetic outflow while enhancing vagal efferents. This results in lower heart rate, decreased heart contractility, lower peripheral arteriolar resistance, and lower venous tone, all of which tend to bring the arterial pressure back down to normal. Conversely, when the pressure becomes too low, decreased baroreceptor firing causes increased sympathetic and decreased vagal outflow, resulting in a higher heart rate, increased heart contractility, higher peripheral arteriolar resistance, and higher venous tone, all tending to elevate blood pressure.

This is a quickly responding system, acting within a heartbeat or two. It therefore works fine in acute situations requiring moment-to-moment adjustment of blood pressure. It is not so effective when compensating for long-term circulatory derangements, such as essential hypertension (high blood pressure).

Venous Baroreceptors

On the venous or "volume" side of the circulation, large volumes will stretch another set of receptors located near the venoatrial junctions. These venous baroreceptors have equivocal effects on the rapidly acting circulatory variables already discussed, but are known to be important in the inherently slower renal regulation of circulating blood volume. The details of how they work are best studied along with renal physiology itself.

MAJOR PHYSICAL PROPERTIES OF THE SYSTEM

We want to emphasize certain physical properties of the circulatory system at this point. Most of the values given for flow and pressure below are worth memorizing.

Flow

The quantity of blood flowing through the aortic valve is called the cardiac output. Flow is usually designated as $\dot{Q}$ (quantity per time), and in a normal adult human, this $\dot{Q}_T$ or total flow is approximately 5 L/min. Although 5 L/min flows through the "root" of the aorta, it splits into separate smaller flows to perfuse each of the various organs. One set of organs, the kidneys, gets a full 20–25% of this flow at rest, far in excess of metabolic need. The kidneys manage to obtain about a liter per minute even during exercise. Because the lungs are arranged in series with the other organs instead of in parallel, the entire 5 L/min cardiac output normally perfuses them.

Total Cross-Sectional Area

The cross-sectional area of the average human aorta is about 4.5 cm². This is the smallest cross-sectional area at any point in the circulation and is illustrated in Fig. 1.3.

Cutting across **every** arteriole and adding up all the cross-sectional areas involved would give a total area of about 400 cm², or roughly 100 times the total area at the aortic level. Repeating this procedure again at the mid-capillary level would yield approximately 4,500 cm², a further increase in area. Blood then flows through the venules into the vena cavas, whose total cross-sectional area is perhaps 18 cm².

Linear Blood Velocities

Cross-sectional circulatory areas help in the understanding of how rapidly (or slowly) blood traverses the different parts of the circulation (Fig. 1.4). For example, the fastest velocities are found in the aorta because the entire flow (5,000 cm³/min) must pass through the narrowest orifice (4.5 cm² area). This calculates out to a speed of 5,000/4.5 = 1,111 cm/min or 185 mm/sec. At the arteriolar level there is a much smaller calculated velocity: 2.1 mm/sec, because of the larger cross-sectional area through which the 5 L/min is flowing. When flowing through the capillaries, blood

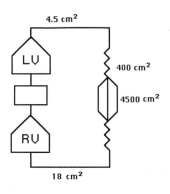

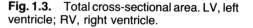

Fig. 1.3. Total cross-sectional area. LV, left ventricle; RV, right ventricle.

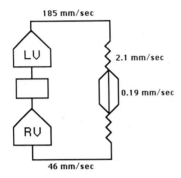

Fig. 1.4. Blood velocity. LV, left ventricle; RV, right ventricle.

is streaming still more slowly at roughly 0.19 mm/sec [= (5,000 cm^3/min)(1 min/60 sec)(10 mm/cm)/(4,500 cm^2)]. Since capillaries are a millimeter or so in length, individual red cells have plenty of time to exchange O_2 and CO_2 with the tissues. Vena caval velocities calculate out to 46 mm/sec. Velocities within the capillary bed of the lungs are similar to those in tissue capillaries, usually giving ample time for the exchange of O_2 and CO_2 to take place.

Pressures

What pressure gradients drive the blood through the circulation? Figure 1.5 summarizes the story, for a recumbent subject, giving

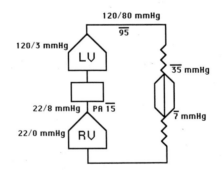

Fig. 1.5. Pressures. LV, left ventricle; RV, right ventricle.

mean pressures as $\overline{95}$ mm Hg for example, and systolic/diastolic pressures as "120/80" mm Hg. The highest pressure in the circulation is found in the left ventricle: 120 mm Hg, developed during systolic ejection. During ventricular relaxation the diastolic pressure falls to a low level, given here as 3 mm Hg. Because the aortic valve closes during ventricular relaxation, the pressure in the aorta doesn't fall as low as ventricular pressure does, and it declines to only 80 mm Hg or so before being increased again by the next systolic ejection from the ventricle. The average aortic pressure is approximately $\overline{95}$ mm Hg, closer to the diastolic value of 80 mm Hg than to the systolic of 120 mm Hg, because the aortic pressure peaks at 120 mm Hg for only a short period of time.

The largest pressure gradient in the circulation occurs "across" the systemic arterioles, where a drop of 60 mm Hg is common. The mean pressure at the distal end of the arterioles, that which perfuses the capillary bed, is thus approximately $\overline{35}$ mm Hg. No systolic or diastolic pressures are given here, because blood pressure and flow have been damped by the combination of aortic distensibility (compliance) and arteriolar resistance. A further pressure drop of 25 mm Hg or more occurs across the capillary bed, to a level of 7 mm Hg or so, as the venules are entered. Even lower pressures are found as the blood flows through the large veins into the right atrium, where negative (subatmospheric) pressures are commonly encountered. Pulsatile values occur again in the great veins, because pressure waves generated by the right atrium and right ventricle are transmitted backward into the venous system.

Typical pressures in the right ventricle are 22/0 mm Hg, and in the pulmonary artery 22/8 mm Hg, with a mean there of approximately $\overline{15}$ mm Hg. The pressure drop across the lung is much smaller than that across the systemic circuit, even though the flow through the lung is substantially the same as that perfusing the rest of the tissues. This is due to a lower vascular resistance in the lung. The average pulmonary venous (i.e., left atrial) pressure is usually slightly higher than comparable pressures on the right side of the circulation, and is approximately 4 mm Hg. This means that in this case the pressure gradient perfusing the lung is

$\overline{15} - \overline{4}$, or only 11 mm Hg, compared to $\overline{95} - \overline{0}$, or 95 mm Hg, perfusing the systemic circulation.

Volumes

The total amount of blood in a human is approximately 8% of body weight. Since the density of blood is close to 1 g/ml, a 72-kg person will have a blood volume of approximately 5.8 L. Figure 1.6 shows a rough picture of how this blood volume is distributed to the parts of the circulation already discussed. Note that the distribution figures vary rather widely from text to text, though there is agreement on the overall picture.

The left ventricle at end diastole will hold something like 125 ml of blood or roughly 2% of the total blood volume. The entire arterial system, though high in pressure, is low in volume at 10% of the total. The arterioles, though they are myriad in number, contain only 1% or so of the volume. The even more numerous capillaries have perhaps 5% of the total. The veins plus right atrium have the lion's share of the circulating volume: 55% or more of the total. After the right ventricle, which holds only 2% of the total, there is another large blood pool in the lungs plus left atrium. Thus about 80% of the blood volume is held in the venous and lung reservoirs. Because the sizes of these reservoirs are under physiologic control, as will be discussed later, these pools of blood

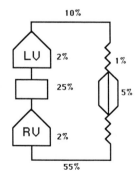

Fig. 1.6. Volumes. LV, left ventricle; RV, right ventricle.

can be effectively ''transfused'' into the arteries to maintain perfusing pressure should the need arise.

Note that the resting flow in liters per minute is almost numerically equal to the total blood volume in liters. This indicates that it should take the average red blood cell roughly 1 min to make the complete circuit. When a person is exercising and the cardiac output is elevated, however, a particular red cell may pass through the aorta three to four times per minute.

Stroke Volume

Cardiac stroke volume is the volume of blood put out per heart beat. Left ventricular and right ventricular stroke volumes, approximately 75 ml at rest, are necessarily equal over even short periods of time, otherwise the blood would pile up in the lungs or in the systemic circulation. The Frank–Starling mechanism is responsible for maintaining this equality, and will be discussed at length later. In certain congenital heart abnormalities there is shunting of blood between heart chambers or between the great vessels, with the result that right and left ventricular stroke volumes may not be equal. (How to calculate these shunts and stroke volumes is discussed in later sections.) Normally left ventricular cardiac output ($\dot{Q}_{LV}$) is equal to the product of heart rate (HR) and left ventricular stroke volume (SV), or

$$\dot{Q} = HR \times SV \qquad [1.1]$$

As the physics of the body unfolds in this introductory text, a multiplicity of such relationships will arise. They are merely compact representations of how the body functions.

Another simple yet important relationship can be found in the definition of stroke volume as the difference between end diastolic volume (EDV) and end systolic volume (ESV):

$$SV = EDV - ESV \qquad [1.2]$$

End diastolic ventricular volume represents the largest volume that the chamber contains before it contracts. End systolic volume is the smallest volume of blood that remains when the heart has stopped contracting.

Pulse Pressure

Pulse pressure is usually important only in the arterial circulations, and is defined as the difference between the systolic or highest arterial pressure, Pa_{sys}, and the diastolic or lowest arterial pressure, Pa_{dias}:

$$P_{pulse} = Pa_{sys} - Pa_{dias} \qquad [1.3]$$

The modifying symbol "a" is on loan from the pulmonary physiologists, who use it to represent "arterial" as opposed to "A" which represents Alveolar. The magnitude of the pulse pressure reflects the distensibility of the arteries, and the size of the stroke volume. How this happens is described later.

STARTING THE SYSTEM

As an exercise to help understand how blood is moved from one part of the circulation to the next, the system will be examined with the pumps turned off and then again after they have been turned back on. The approach here follows the lead of Arthur Guyton whose textbooks make frequent use of similiar physical models.

The Circulation at Rest

Although it will rarely if ever occur in a healthy animal, what would happen to pressures in the circulation if the heart suddenly stopped? Assuming that one could have a look before reflex changes took place (slightly unrealistic), and before fluid could leak between vessels and surroundings (relatively realistic), what pressures would be measured at various points around the circuit in a supine animal? Guyton claims, and many others are inclined to agree, that under such circumstances blood will flow readily between the connected vessels until pressure is the same everywhere within the vascular system. In experiments in which the heart has been electrically arrested or in others in which flow has been stopped by inflating balloon catheters at selected points, this so-called ''mean circulatory pressure'' has been found to be approximately 7–10 mm Hg. Mean circulatory pressure can also be conceived as the pressure that would result from filling a previously empty circulation with a normal blood volume, being careful to maintain a normal vascular tone. This last restriction is not physiologically reasonable and makes this conceptual filling experiment impossible on a practical level.

The largest and most distensible compartment in the circulation is the venules plus veins, where the pressure is normally about 7–10 mm Hg even before shutting off the pumps. The fluid shift from high-pressure, stiff arteries into low-pressure, compliant veins will produce a large fall in arterial pressure, but a negligible rise in venous pressure.

This means that even under extreme conditions, if vascular tone and circulatory volume are held constant, the mean circulatory pressure residing in the large venular reservoir remains constant. This gives an important, reasonably constant reference point within the circulation. Hereafter, for pedagogical purposes, think of the venular (mean circulatory) pressure as being **unaffected** in a direct way by the pumps, but subject to change by shifts in blood volume and venous tone.

This is an oversimplification, but a good first-order approximation to how the circulation works. Older textbooks do not discuss it, and many recent texts treat the idea of mean circulatory pressure cursorily or even incorrectly. The trend, however, is toward acceptance, if only because it makes it easier to teach how the circulation works. Physiology texts and papers are full of simple models, none of which works all the time. Usually, a successful physiologist or a successful physician will choose a model appropriate to the situation being studied, and will be willing to ignore complicating but second-order effects.

The Circulation in Action

What happens in all those vascular compartments once comfortably resting at 7 mm Hg pressure when the heart starts beating? Consider the pulmonary artery, which is suddenly receiving extra blood at its ventricular end. It has but a limited compliance (stretchability) and only narrow, high-resistance pipes out of which blood can leak. As the steady state is being achieved, its pressure rises from 7 to 15 mm Hg. The extra blood causing this pressure rise comes from the right atrium and great veins. The pressure in these structures falls from 7 to near 0 mm Hg. There will be little or no change in venular pressure (still near 7 mm Hg). It is mainly the pressure gradient of 7 mm Hg in the large venular reservoir to near 0 mm Hg in the right atrium that causes the blood to flow from venules to right atrium once these pumps are turned on. Note that since these pressures remain unequal during the resulting steady state, we have to deduce the existence of a "venous resistance" between venules and right atrium.

The same sort of thing will happen on the systemic side of the circulation. An equal quantity of blood is moved from easily stretchable pulmonary veins to very stiff arteries out of which blood exits with some difficulty. The result is a small fall in pulmonary venous–left atrial pressure (from 7 to 3–4 mm Hg) and a large rise in aortic pressure (from 7 to 95 mm Hg). The pressure gradient (95 − 7 mm Hg) drives blood through the systemic (arteriolar plus capillary) resistance.

SUMMARY

The main and immediate purpose of the circulation is to perfuse the brain, heart, and lungs at all costs. It does this by maintaining arterial blood pressure at reasonable levels, sacrificing flow through lesser organs if necessary. Over the short term, the body is kept informed through an intelligence network known as the arterial baroreceptor system. Signals from the baroreceptors are integrated in medullary centers within the central nervous system, and produce output signals via the sympathetics and vagus. These signals stimulate or inhibit four important circulatory control mechanisms. These are:

1. Heart rate
2. Ventricular contractility
3. Arteriolar resistance
4. Venous tone

The first two determine cardiac output, the third offers opposition to the flow of blood between arteries and capillaries in order to maintain general arterial pressure, and the fourth helps to push blood from the venous reservoir into the right atrium. Sympathetic efferents thus increase heart rate, heart contractility, arteriolar resistance, and venous tone, while vagal efferents lower heart rate and have little or no well-documented effects on other circulatory variables.

Each anatomic portion of the circulation has individual characteristics. The arteries comprise a relatively stiff, low-volume distribution system in which circulatory energy is stored at high pressure for continuous release during the cardiac cycle. The arterioles are the resistive faucets that keep up the arterial pressure while determining how much blood flow individual tissues will be allotted. Capillaries have both a large cross-sectional area and a large lateral surface area for gas and nutrient exchange with adjacent tissues. The blood flows through them at very slow linear velocities. The veins and venules act as a huge, easily distensible blood reservoir, and serve as low pressure conduits that bring blood back to the pumps for redistribution.

QUESTIONS

1.01. The mean linear velocity of a red blood cell will be lowest in the:

a. Elastic arteries.
b. Large veins.
c. Right ventricle.
d. Capillaries.
e. Arterioles.

1.02. An increase in carotid sinus discharge causes a reflex increase in:

a. Activity in sympathetic vasoconstrictor nerves.
b. Activity in vagal efferent nerves going to the heart.
c. Cardiac force of contraction.
d. Heart rate.
e. Venous tone.

1.03. Of the following, the right and left ventricles differ most in their:

a. Response to cardiac sympathetic nerve activity.
b. Inflow of venous blood per minute.
c. Output of blood per minute.
d. Work performed per minute.
e. Average stroke volume.

Questions 1.04–1.07 refer to a recumbent subject. Choose from a–e below in answering the next four questions.

a. Systemic arteries.
b. Systemic arterioles.
c. Systemic capillaries.
d. Systemic venules.
e. Systemic veins.

1.04. Taken together, which two of the listed vessel types contain the largest volume of blood under normal circumstances?

1.05. Which of the listed vessels, considered individually, usually has the largest radius?

1.06. If all the vessels that operate in parallel are added together, which listed vessel type has the greatest cross-sectional area?

1.07. From beginning to end of which of the listed vessels does the largest fall in pressure take place?

1.08. What are the definitions of arterial systolic, diastolic, and mean pressures? How can they be measured? What are their values in normal resting humans?

Although we stress problem solving in physiology, we still want you to remember some normal physiological values. Try to give the important figures for resting humans in **Questions 1.09–1.14.**

1.09. What are the normal values for P_{O_2} in systemic arteries and in systemic veins?

1.10. What are the normal values for O_2 content in systemic arteries and in systemic veins?

1.11. What are the normal values for P_{CO_2} in systemic arteries and systemic veins?

1.12. What is the normal value for O_2 consumption ($\dot{V}_{O_2}$)?

1.13. What is the normal value for CO_2 production ($\dot{V}_{CO_2}$)?

1.14. What is the normal value for cardiac output ($\dot{Q}$)?

ANSWERS

1.01. d. The same blood flow, $\dot{Q}$, must be coursing through the arteries, arterioles, capillaries, venules, and veins, as these segments are arranged in series with one another. However, the cross-sectional area is smallest at the aorta, increases by perhaps a thousandfold by the time one reaches the capillaries, and then decreases greatly again by the time one arrives at the vena cavae. Thus, the linear velocity of each red cell must be greatest at the aorta and smallest at the capillaries.

1.02. b. The physiological event which would normally cause an increase in carotid sinus discharge is an increase in arterial blood pressure. The reflex mechanisms must be designed, therefore, to bring the pressure back down. Alternative b will do this by slowing the heart rate. All other choices will tend to increase the blood pressure.

1.03. d. The two ventricles have the same $\dot{Q}_{in}$, $\dot{Q}_{out}$, heart rate, and stroke volume. Both respond to sympathetic stimulation by increasing their force of contraction. However, the right ventricle drives blood through the low resistance pulmonary circulation, while the left must supply the higher resistance systemic circulation. The work of the left ventricle is five or more times that of the right because the mean aortic pressure is five or more times that in the pulmonary artery.

1.04. d,e.

1.05. e.

1.06. c.

1.07. b.

1.08. Arterial systolic and diastolic pressures are the highest and the lowest pressures, respectively, that occur in the arteries. Typical values are 120 and 80 mm Hg. They are most commonly measured noninvasively with a sphygmomanometer. Alternatively, in experimental animals and in hospitalized patients, a liquid-filled tube can be inserted into an artery and connected to a mercury manometer or to a pressure transducer. Mean arterial pressure is the average arterial pressure during the cardiac cycle, commonly about 95 mm Hg. Obtaining an accurate value requires dealing with time–pressure areas, and is usually done electronically.

1.09. $Pa_{O_2} = 90 - 100$ mm Hg. $P\bar{v}_{O_2} = 40$ mm Hg.

1.10. Ca_{O_2} = 200 ml O_2/L blood. $C\bar{V}_{O_2}$ = 150 ml O_2/L blood.

1.11. Pa_{CO_2} = 40 mm Hg. $P\bar{V}_{CO_2}$ = 46 mm Hg.

1.12. For a basal 70-kg male, $\dot{V}_{O_2}$ = 250 ml O_2/min, STPD.

1.13. For a basal 70-kg male, $\dot{V}_{CO_2}$ = 200 ml O_2/min, STPD.

1.14. For a resting 70-kg male, $\dot{Q}$ = 5–5.5 L blood/min.

2

Electrical Aspects of the Heart

INTRODUCTION

This section will give some understanding of (1) how transmembrane ion fluxes in heart muscle cells are related to transmembrane electrical potentials, (2) how changes in these transmembrane potentials produce electrocardiographic (EKG) potential changes at the body surface, and (3) how a few of the common abnormalities of this system can be diagnosed using the EKG. A brief sketch of cardiac electrophysiology is presented, followed by a simplified development of the EKG and short discussions of some common EKG disturbances.

CARDIAC CELLULAR ELECTROPHYSIOLOGY

Membrane Resting Potential

Even "resting" (not contracting at the moment) cardiac muscle cells maintain an electrical potential difference across their cell plasma membranes. In mammalian ventricular cells this may range from -70 mV to -85 mV, where the inside of such resting cells is negatively charged with respect to the outside. Cell membranes are maintained in this "polarized" state by the Na^+ pump.

The "Na^+ pump" is a Na^+/K^+ exchange pump which trades Na^+ for K^+ in such a way that Na^+ is pumped out of the cell at the same time that K^+ is pumped in. The trade is approximately 3 Na^+ out for each 2 K^+ in, so that the pump is electrogenic (produces a membrane potential). The following section ignores this contribution to the resting membrane potential and concentrates on the quantitatively more important contributions of ionic gradients produced by the Na^+/K^+ pump.

Special Case of Membrane Equilibrium—The Nernst Potential

Whereas a **steady state** requires continual energy input for maintenance, a true **equilibrium** represents a static balance of forces with no ongoing ion or energy flows through the system. The resting cell membrane is **almost** in this latter state. Consider the cell in Fig. 2.1. Assume it is capable of reaching an equilibrium state and has the following properties:

1. It has preset, fixed ionic gradients with its intracellular fluid high in K^+ and low in Na^+ and Ca^{2+}, and it has an extracellular fluid low in K^+ but rich in Na^+ and Ca^{2+}.
2. It is leaky *only* to K^+.

One might assume that because $[K]_{in} > [K]_{out}$, most of the K^+ would leak out of the cell. But before **half of 1%** of cellular K^+ has left the cell, the leak stops. If the cell had had a glycerol leak instead of a K^+ leak, the glycerol would have continued to leak out. As K^+ starts to leak out, however, it leaves unsatisfied negative

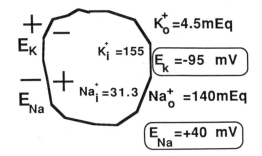

FIG. 2.1. Generation of the Nernst membrane potential.

charges behind (principally anionic proteins, lipids, and some phosphates and chloride). The K^+ leak thus sets up an electrical field which acts to make the exit of subsequent cations progressively more difficult. The net result is that while cellular ionic concentrations are not measureably changed, the inside of the cell has become negatively charged with respect to the outside. An equilibrium has been established between **chemical concentration forces** tending to push K^+ out of the cell and **electrical forces** tending just as hard to push K^+ back into the cell.

The equation describing this **Nernst equilibrium potential** is a statement that these forces are balanced for K^+:

$$E_{K^+} = (RT/F) \ln(K]_{out}/[K]_{in})$$

or, at 37°C:

$$E_{K^+} = 61.5 \log_{10}([K]_{out}/[K]_{in}) \text{ mV} \qquad [2.1]$$

61.5 is the millivolt equivalence of RT/F, where R is the Universal gas constant, T is the absolute temperature and F is the Faraday. Equation 2.1 is important enough that we ask you to memorize it. If the pictured cell membrane were leaky only to K^+, and if the inside and outside K^+ concentrations (really activities) were 155 and 4.5 mEq, respectively, the equilibrium membrane potential would be -95 mV. What this relationship says is that -95 mV is the **electrical** equivalent of a 4.5/155 **concentration** gradient of K^+.

Now suppose that the membrane were leaky to Na^+ instead of K^+. What would happen? Some Na^+ (a chemically trivial amount) would leak inward, charging the inside positive with respect to the outside. If such a Na^+ leak were present with the Na^+ concentrations pictured, the cell's electrical potential would be given by the Nernst relation as:

$$E_{Na^+} = 61.5 \log_{10}(140/31.3) = +40 \text{ mV}$$

In other words, merely switching from a K^+ leak to a Na^+ leak would completely change the cell's electrical picture from a negatively polarized state to a positively polarized state.

Real Life, the Steady State, and the Goldman Potential

Although cardiac ventricular cells have a high K conductance (g_K, K^+ leak) in their resting state, they are just a tad leaky to Na^+ and other ions as well. Using assumptions about membrane potential profiles that we shall not go into here, David Goldman formulated an equation that describes the living steady state reasonably well:

$$E_M = 61.5 \log_{10} \frac{P_K[K]_{out} + P_{Na}[Na]_{out} + P_{Cl}[Cl]_{in}}{P_K[K]_{in} + P_{Na}[Na]_{in} + P_{Cl}[Cl]_{out}} \quad [2.2]$$

In this equation the P values stand for permeability to potassium, etc., and E_M is in millivolts. Ca^{2+} and other ions have been left out for simplicity. One should be able to see from this equation that when the membrane is very leaky to K^+ and not at all to anything else (i.e., $P_K > P_{Na}$ and P_{Cl}), the Goldman equation reduces to the Nernst K equilibrium relationship. Again, note that ionic permeabilities (or ionic conductances) can control membrane potentials.

In this steady-state, nonequilibrium situation, the whole system would eventually run down if energy were not being supplied in some form. At any reasonable resting membrane potential, no ion would be exactly at equilibrium and hence all ions would be leaking. This would be a real mess, except that the Na/K exchange pump opposes the Na and K leaks and maintains their ionic gradients quite nicely. A separate Ca^{2+} pump picks up loose ends in the Ca^{2+} department. Cl^- seems to have no pump of its own in cardiac muscle cells, and so its ionic gradient simply passively reflects the average existing membrane potential. The K permeabilities of cardiac ventricular muscle cells at rest are so much higher than their Na permeabilities that their resting potentials (about -85 mV) are quite close to the calculated potassium equilibrium potential (about -95 mV) representing their concentration gradients. Resting ventricular cells are thus said to approximate "potassium electrodes" in that their potentials accurately reflect the K concentration of the fluid they sit in.

Membrane Action Potential

While many of our cells seem content with the ionic and electrical potential gradients imposed on them by the ion pumps and fixed ion leaks already described, nerve and muscle cells are different. Through mechanisms poorly understood at the molecular level, these cells are capable of modifying their membrane ion permeabilities in response to signals from neighboring cells so as to create time-varying or "action" potentials across the cell membrane. In the heart, these action potentials then encourage other contiguous cells to engage in the same process, resulting in the propagation of an electrical response throughout the tissue. Figure 2.2 is a schematic picture of the transmembrane electrical potential changes that occur in a typical ventricular cell. The resting potential of -85 mV (inside negative) is similar to that of other body cells, but the sudden upstroke is what makes it different. There is strong evidence that in cardiac muscle cells, as in nerves, a sudden increase in Na^+ conductance ($g_{Na,fast}$) in the "fast sodium channels" and a fall in K conductance (g_K) drive the membrane potential toward the Na^+ equilibrium potential, so that the membrane potential be-

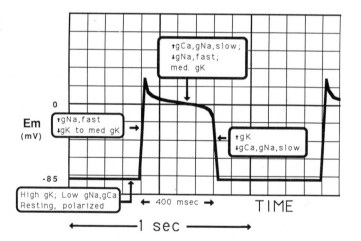

FIG. 2.2. Transmembrane action potential in a ventricular muscle cell.

comes transiently positive. This shift away from the resting or polarized state is often called depolarization, even though the resulting potential may leave the membrane in a slightly positively or negatively polarized condition. This is followed by an immediate fall in $g_{Na,fast}$ and a rise in both g_{Ca} and slow sodium channel conductance ($g_{Na,slow}$), stabilizing the membrane potential for a time in the so-called "plateau" phase. During this important part of the action potential the relatively high g_{Ca} allows Ca^{2+} to flow down its electrochemical potential gradient from outside to inside the cell where it triggers mechanical contraction. A subsequent fall in g_{Ca} and rise in g_K restore the membrane potential to its resting negative value, and the cell awaits the next signal from its neighbor to repeat the entire process. The events in nerve and skeletal muscle cells are similar, except that such cells lack the prolonged period of calcium influx, and their action potentials are therefore considerably shorter in duration. Calcium for the contractile units of skeletal muscle derives principally from the sarcoplasmic reticulum which is more abundant in that tissue. The sarcoplasmic reticulum within cardiac muscle cells probably does contribute a portion of the calcium required for contraction.

Pacemaker Cells (SA Node)

The sinoatrial (SA) node is a small group of specialized muscle cells lying in the posterior superior wall of the right atrium. Within this node lie pacemaker cells which generate action potentials that determine the heart rate. They differ from ordinary cardiac muscle cells in that they have an unstable resting potential which drifts slowly in a positive direction (Fig. 2.3) until a threshold value is reached. At this point g_{Na} increases, causing a more rapid depolarization of the cell. This slow drift is referred to as a slow diastolic depolarization, or as the prepotential phase of the action potential, and is probably due to a slow decrease of g_K.

Action potentials of pacemaker cells also lack the Ca^{2+} plateau phase, which is consistent with the function of these cells as generators of electrical signals rather than actively contracting units. In

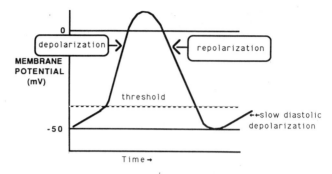

FIG. 2.3. Membrane potential of a normal pacemaker cell.

a normal physiological setting it is likely that only one pacemaker cell in the SA node, the most rapidly depolarizing one, actually goes through this spontaneous process all the way to completion. Its neighbors, because they are slower on the uptake, never reach threshold on their own before they are told by an adjacent cell what to do.

Control of Heart Rate

This is an appropriate place to discuss the control of heart rate, because the slow diastolic depolarization phase of SA node cells offers the key. Figure 2.4 depicts some of the changes to be seen. Increased efferent activity from the vagus slows heart rate both by slowing the rate at which diastolic depolarization rises and by making the resting membrane potential more negative (not shown), thus decreasing the frequency with which a pacemaker cell reaches threshold in a given period of time. An increase in sympathetic tone or a decrease in vagal tone acts in the opposite way to increase pacemaker frequency by shortening the time taken to reach threshold. These actions are consistent with the roles played in the circulation by the vagus and sympathetics: The vagus acts as a brake, and the sympathetics as an accelerator. Hormones and drugs also act by this mechanism. From Fig. 2.4 one can see that the length of

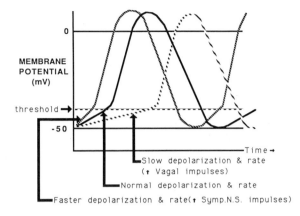

FIG. 2.4. Autonomic nervous system effects on membrane potential of normal pacemaker cell.

an action potential and the level of the threshold potential must also be important in determining heart rate. How these latter variables are controlled is beyond the scope of this discussion, however.

THE CONDUCTION SYSTEM

Cell-to-Cell Conduction

The periodic signals of the SA nodal pacemaker are propagated from cell to cell throughout the heart (Fig. 2.5) by way of gap junctions, regions of cell membrane contact that have low electrical resistance. Within the atria this excitation wave spreads rapidly via atrial muscle cells themselves, although there is some evidence for preferential pathways in the atrial walls. As each atrial cell produces an action potential, Ca^{2+} soon becomes available to its contractile units, and both atria contract in unison. Contraction always lags behind electrical depolarization, because both ionic diffusion and biochemical reactions intervene between the electrical and mechanical processes.

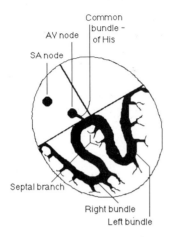

FIG. 2.5. Electrical conduction system. AV, atrioventricular; SA, sinoatrial.

The Atrioventricular Node

After traversing the atrial muscle, the excitation wave enters a specialized, slowly conducting region known as the atrioventricular (AV) node. The normal conduction delay in this structure allows the atria to get on with contraction before the ventricles leap into action. The AV node thereby offers a point for the autonomic nervous system to control ventricular responses to atrial depolarizations. Increasing vagal efferent activity slows conduction through the AV node, and conversely, increasing sympathetic activity speeds impulse transmission to the ventricles. Hormones and drugs also have access to this same mechanism, with acetylcholine mimicking vagal effects, and norepinephrine mimicking sympathetic effects. Note that these effects on the AV node assure that when the **SA** node is stimulated to produce faster heart rates, the **AV** node will transmit the impulses at a faster velocity. The reader should note carefully that under normal circumstances heart rate is **not** controlled via the AV node.

The His–Purkinje System

From the AV node, the excitation wave enters the ventricular septum via the common bundle of His, part of a rapidly conducting pathway, the His–Purkinje system, which traverses the entire ventricular endocardium (Fig. 2.5). The anatomically small common bundle of His is normally the only pathway by which the excitation signal passes through the otherwise fibrous, nonmuscular annulus that separates atria from ventricles. Purkinje cells closely resemble ventricular muscle cells in microstructure but are richer in glycogen and poorer in contractile units. Within a few millimeters, the common bundle splits into right and left bundle branches which proceed along the endocardial surface to the apex, where a network of finer branches then spread to the ventricular ''bases'' across the remainder of the endocardial surface of the free ventricular walls. Even finer branches from these endocardial fibers then penetrate the ventricular muscle for varying depths. The interventricular septum is most often innervated by early twigs from the left bundle, a fact of some diagnostic importance. This often causes depolarization to proceed earlier in the septum than elsewhere in the ventricles, and in a left-to-right direction. It should be emphasized that transmission through the His–Purkinje system is so rapid that the onset of depolarization in the remaining ventricular endocardium is almost simultaneous. The excitation wave then spreads more slowly from endocardium to epicardium through the ventricular muscle cells themselves. Good evidence indicates that the Purkinje system penetrates through a portion of the ventricular wall, so that the slower wave of excitation within the muscle has a consistent outward direction only in the outer third of the wall.

FROM ACTION POTENTIAL TO THE EKG

Assumptions About Dipoles and Excitation Pathways

The physicist–physician Hermann Helmholtz proved conclusively in 1853 that it is impossible to deduce solely from potential distributions on the surface of a body the nature of the electrical generators inside that body. Undaunted, physicians, physiologists, and textbooks continue to explain how the EKG describes the electrical state of the myocardium. This text is no exception to this common practice. However, we need add but a few assumptions to produce a scheme that would be equally acceptable to Helmholtz, to the bedside physician, and to the beginning physiology student.

We begin by assuming that at any instant in time the effect of all transmembrane potentials in the heart can be represented as a single-charge dipole located within the thorax. For our purposes only the orientation and relative magnitude of this dipole will be important. By further attributing a particular time sequence of dipole orientations and magnitudes to a particular activation sequence within the heart, we will be in a position to explain basic electrical pathology.

The Depolarization Pattern

Figure 2.6 shows what we expect to find when recording electrical potentials externally (not in a transmembrane fashion) from a single ventricular cell or a large ensemble of electrically connected cells. Fig. 2.6a shows a resting cell with negative transmembrane potential represented by an excess of negative charge within the cell and an excess of positive charge without. This charge distribution can be represented by a series of small electrical dipoles symmetrically located around the cell membrane. Because of this symmetry recording electrodes placed at a respectable distance away from the cell (>10 μm) measure a zero electrical field or zero potential difference between the electrodes. The **transmembrane** potential difference, nevertheless, is approximately -85 mV at the same time. As the depolarization process moves down the cell membrane from left to right, however, there will be a nonsymmetrical charge distribution when the left portion of the cell membrane has been depolarized to the plateau phase (near zero membrane potential) and the right portion is still in the resting state (-85 mV; Fig. 2.6b). If we consider that the plateau occurs at a zero or small positive transmembrane potential, then we can see that the dipoles in the left (shaded) portion of the cell will no longer balance the dipoles of the right, and a net cellular electrical dipole will exist. We take the direction of this dipole arbitrarily to point to the positive charge, i.e., to the right in this figure. Extracellular electrodes will sense an electrical potential difference between the left and right ends of the cell,

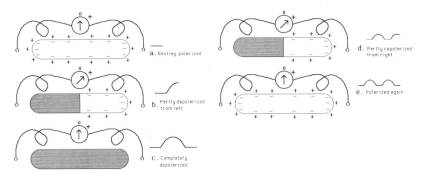

FIG. 2.6. Pattern of depolarization.

and by convention, an associated potentiometer (sensitive voltmeter) will give a positive reading (see Table 2.1). Electrocardiographic systems are arbitrarily wired to produce a positive or upright deflection when the so-called positive or exploring electrode is at a higher or more positive potential than the so-called negative or reference electrode.

TABLE 2.1. *Electrocardiographic leads*

Limb leads			Chest leads[a]	
Name	Record deflects upward when this electrode is more positive than its mate.	Record reflects downward when this electrode is more positive than its mate.	Name	Exploring electrode
I	left arm	right arm	V1	Right sternal border in 4th interspace
II	left leg	right arm	V2	Left sternal border in 4th interspace
III	left leg	left arm	V3	Halfway between V2 and V4
aVR	right arm	left arm and left leg	V4	Midclavicular line in 5th interspace
aVL	left arm	right arm and left leg	V5	Anterior axillary line at same horizontal level as V4
aVF	left leg	right arm and left arm	V6	Mid axillary line at same horizontal level as V4

[a] A reference electrode is wired simultaneously to the left and right arms and the left leg. When the exploring electrode listed below is more positive than this reference electrode, there is an upright deflection.

Such an asymmetry will persist only during the brief time that the upstroke of the action potential is actually traversing this cell. When the entire cell membrane reaches the plateau phase the charge distribution will again appear symmetrical to external electrodes, and a potential of zero will again be recorded externally (Fig. 2.6c). Thus, while the transmembrane potentials of this cell may be quite different from those found at rest (Figs. 2.6a and 2.6c), pairs of outside electrodes will see zero potential difference. This is a cogent demonstration of Helmholtz's principle enunciated earlier, that different internal electrical generators can produce identical external effects.

The Repolarization Pattern

If life is to go on, repolarization must follow depolarization, and the cell membrane must return to its resting state. In human left ventricles this happens in a curious way: Epicardial cells and the epicardial ends of the remaining cells tend to repolarize before endocardial cells do, even though these epicardial regions are usually the last to depolarize. Contrary to this pattern, heart muscle strips, skeletal muscle strips, and the intact hearts of small animals exhibit the expected sequence of first depolarized, first repolarized. It is thought that the later repolarization of the endocardial region in human ventricles is related to the development of higher local myocardial wall stress. Consequently, we have depicted a partially repolarized cell in Fig. 2.6d with external electrodes showing a positive reading again as the asymmetrical dipoles once more point to the right.

When the entire cell has returned to the resting or polarized state (Fig. 2.6e), a zero external potential reading returns. A schematic recording of the entire ventricular activation cycle is shown at the right of each part of Fig. 2.6. Note that both the depolarization and repolarization processes produce positive dipole components on these recordings. Be aware that extracellular recordings of **atrial** potentials will often indicate depolarization and repolarization dipoles pointing in opposite directions.

Electrocardiographic Conventions

When instead of a single heart cell we have the whole heart, and instead of small electrodes we have electrodes affixed to various bodily parts, we say we are taking an EKG, but we continue to analyze the record as above. The EKG often looks like Fig. 2.7a. A simultaneously inscribed transmembrane potential of a single ventricular cell might look like Fig. 2.7b. In analyzing such EKG tracings we assume that the wave identified as ''P'' represents atrial depolarization, and that atrial repolarization usually takes place during ventricular depolarization (QRS complex), and is not present as a separate wave. The ''T'' wave we associate with ventricular repolarization. In healthy individuals it usually points, as it does in Fig. 2.7, in the net direction of the QRS.

The naming convention for EKG waves is arbitrary. P and T waves can be upright, biphasic, or inverted. If ventricular depolarization commences with a downward deflection, it is a Q wave. The first upward deflection of the QRS is an R wave, and the first downward deflection following an R is an S wave. A second upward deflection is called an R' (R prime), and a second downward deflec-

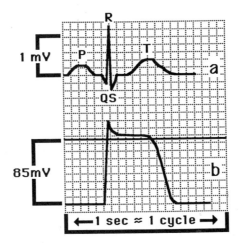

FIG. 2.7. Cardiac electrical activity—extracellular and intracellular.

tion to follow an R is called an S′. Should there be only a downward deflection, with no upward wave present, it is termed a QS. Thus, by definition, R is always up, and Q and S are always down.

Depolarization and Repolarization as Seen on the EKG

Figure 2.8 combines the ideas presented in Figs. 2.5–2.7, and shows the recording of potentials from the whole heart using electrocardiographic leads hooked up to the left and right arms. Positivity in the left arm and negativity in the right (associated with a dipole pointing toward the left arm) will produce an upright deflection in this EKG lead (lead I). In Fig. 2.8 the unshaded areas represent

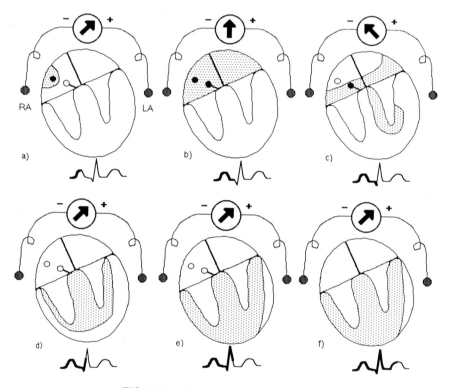

FIG. 2.8. Sequential genesis of EKG.

resting (polarized) atrial and ventricular muscle, and the shaded areas represent depolarized tissue. The six parts of the figure show five snapshots of the spread of the depolarization wave and one of the repolarization process. The dark arrows represent the vector sum of net instantaneous electrical dipoles within the body due to the heart. An externally measurable dipole is absent in at least three situations: (1) in the completely polarized state (resting), (2) in the completely depolarized state, and (3) between atrial and ventricular depolarization (Fig. 2.8b). At other times external electrodes will register potential differences at the body surface. When other muscles are not depolarizing, these potentials are assumed to reflect the strength and orientation of the cardiac net electrical dipole. Thus, as the excitation wave passes from SA to AV node through atrial cells, it will produce a set of small electrical dipoles which appear from a suitably distant vantage point as a composite instantaneous dipole usually pointing toward the legs and the left arm and away from the head and the right arm (Fig. 2.8a).

When atrial cell membranes have all been depolarized, and the excitation process is passing through the small mass of the AV node prior to ventricular activation, there are very few net dipoles being generated. Electrodes external to the heart will record a baseline (zero) potential difference (Fig. 2.8b). Soon after the excitation wave has entered the bundle branches, two electrical events occur: (1) the atria begin to repolarize, generally in the area first depolarized around the SA node, and (2) the interventricular septal muscle cells begin to depolarize from left to right (Fig. 2.8c). Because the atrial mass is relatively small, and because the repolarization process does not happen in a concerted, directed fashion, the atrial repolarization sequence is usually not seen on the EKG. Instead, ventricular depolarization will dominate the electrical picture. Because the ventricular septum is usually supplied from branches of the left bundle of His, septal depolarization from left toward right is often the first part of the ventricular excitation process to be seen by external electrodes. The usual orientation of the net dipole will be away from the left arm and tend to produce a negative deflection in lead I, inscribed here as a Q wave.

Septal depolarization is brief and very soon the mass of ventricular muscle dominates the electrical scene as the depolarization signal is transmitted epicardially by the ramifying Purkinje system (Fig. 2.8d). This produces an instantaneous net dipole pointing toward the feet and the left arm, and hence an upright deflection in lead I. This upright lead I deflection is further enhanced as the right ventricle becomes completely depolarized (electrically silent), and the thicker left ventricle is still being depolarized (Fig. 2.8e). When the entire ventricle has been depolarized (not pictured), there is usually no net dipole, and hence a baseline EKG value is recorded in the so-called ST segment.

In human and other large mammalian hearts, muscle cells nearest the epicardium generally begin their spontaneous repolarization first, producing instantaneous dipoles that usually point in the same direction that the average depolarization dipole had pointed during the QRS. Because the QRS is usually upright in lead I, the T or repolarization wave is usually upright also (Fig. 2.8f). A large disparity in QRS and T dipole vector directions is often a sign of serious cardiac disease.

When all ventricular cells have repolarized back to their resting potentials, no net dipole remains, the heart is electrically silent, and the EKG is once again at baseline.

Some Implications for the EKG

Certain points about the generation of the EKG need emphasis. Most importantly, this external signal is generated only by groups of cells that are actually in the process of depolarizing or repolarizing, and these groups must be large. In contrast, structures as small as the SA or AV node or even the entire His–Purkinje conduction system are usually not electrically visible from the standard surface electrodes of the EKG. Thus, at any given time we can discern only the **boundary** between large masses of resting and activated muscle within the atrial and ventricular walls. Pathology in the conduction system itself will not produce direct effects on the EKG pattern, and will have to be diagnosed from the changes it produces in the de- and repolarization patterns of the heart muscle it serves to activate. Underlying the entire diagnostic process is the assumption that even sick hearts at one time had a normal activation/recovery sequence producing a normal EKG. Lacking this assumption, the body surface potentials can tell us nothing.

EKG LEAD SYSTEMS

The approximately 100-mV swings of transmembrane potential in cardiac muscle cells produce roughly 1-mV changes in potential at the body surface. Although a given patient may lie comfortably in bed many hundreds of volts (not merely millivolts) above ground potential, the small electrocardiographic potential changes are easy to record with modern electronic equipment. Through the years cardiologists have evolved a set of recording leads that have helped us to establish diagnostic criteria for charting the progress of individual patients. The following section describes the common clinical 12-lead system.

The first six leads are usually recorded from combinations of the three electrodes placed on the arms and the left leg. Table 2.1 shows the arrangements. Given only three locations for recording potential and the necessity of measuring potential differences between these points, not absolute potentials, all the electrical information available in the frontal plane of the body can be obtained from any two of the six possible limb leads. Six leads are recorded because this makes it easier to establish the time-average dipole orientation at a glance.

The six-limb leads report cardiac electrical activity occurring in the frontal plane of the body. Figure 2.9 gives two equivalent representations of this hexaxial system: the so-called Einthoven triangle and an older but somehow less traditional Cartesian system. Plotting the standard (I, II, III) and augmented (aVR, aVL, aVF) leads on the same scale is not quite correct, since the former are really enhanced by 15% over the latter. The assumption that electrodes attached to our arms and a leg form an equilateral triangle stretches reality, but we will ignore the error involved. A rule

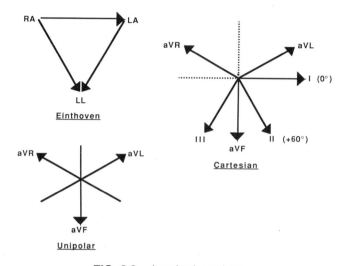

FIG. 2.9. Lead orientations.

that follows from potential theory, no matter what the shape of the triangle, is that at any **instant,** the voltage in lead I plus the voltage in lead III is equal to the voltage in lead II. The same is true for time-average excursions such as the mean QRS voltage in these leads. This relationship (I + III = II) is often referred to as Einthoven's law.

The heart's **net** electrical dipole considered at a particular instant, say part way through ventricular depolarization, will have a spatial magnitude and direction. Usually the orientation of this **instantaneous dipole** will produce a large positive deflection in lead II, since it will be most closely aligned with this lead. Lead aVL, because it is perpendicular to lead II, should experience only a very small deflection, if any.

In the above discussion we have shown how electrical processes in the heart produce electrical potential changes on the surface of the body. The real electrocardiographic problem is the inverse of this. One starts with measured surface electric potentials and tries to figure out what cardiac electrical activity could have caused them. One asks questions like: What is happening when the electrical signal is positive and largest in lead II? If one is allowed the usual assumptions about the depolarization/repolarization history, one usually answers "ventricular depolarization." Without these additional assumptions, the answers could as well have been "the inscription of a very tall T wave in the presence of high serum potassium" or "there is a C battery passing through the patient's esophagus."

The reference system formed by the limb leads can also be used to describe the **time-average or mean dipole vector** associated with, say, ventricular depolarization. To obtain such a measure, one could average all the instantaneous vectors from start to finish of a QRS complex, making use of any two limb leads at a time, and plot the resultant QRS vector. A less accurate but quicker way to get the direction of the mean QRS vector is to look for the lead with the largest R wave and say: "That's the direction of the dipole most of the time." A somewhat better approach, and one that is used clinically, is to look for the lead in which there is essentially no QRS deflection and then assert that the QRS has been pointing perpendicular to this all the while. Since a perpendicular has two possible opposing directions, you will have to exercise a certain amount of clinical judgment here.

Similar determinations can be made of the ventricular repolarization process by measuring the mean axis of the T wave. It usually points in the same direction as the mean QRS in any patient, and deviations often mean disease.

The limb leads do not provide information in the direction of the anteroposterior axis of the body, and this is usually supplied by recording electrical potentials from the anterior chest wall via six chest leads. A turn of the knob on the usual EKG machine to the "V lead" position hooks the reference end of the machine up to both arms and the left leg simultaneously and lets one explore the chest with an electrode as indicated in Table 2.1. Functionally, the reference electrode may be considered to lie just behind the heart. Signals from these chest leads constitute a more or less horizontal electrical section of the body, as opposed to the frontal section presented by the limb leads. Since these electrodes are applied quite close to the heart muscle itself, however, they are influenced strongly by local events. Thus, they report a mixture of net dipole and local news. For example, lead V5 is quite sensitive to left ventricular electrical events, while V1 and V2 are strongly influenced by right ventricular happenings.

EXCITATION–CONTRACTION COUPLING

While membrane action potentials and cardiac contraction are intimately related, they are not the same thing, and it is possible, at least in special situations, to have an EKG tracing without a contraction. Contraction without an EKG signal is harder to come by, however. Thus, the excitation process allows all the myocardial cell membranes to depolarize, sending a wave of Ca^{2+} into the intracellular space during the plateau of the action potential and probably triggering the simultaneous release of a similar wave of Ca^{2+} from sequestered stores in the sarcoplasmic reticulum. Because ionic movements and biochemical reactions link the electrical event to mechanical contraction, there is an inherent lag of perhaps 0.05 sec between the onset of the QRS and the onset of contraction.

These Ca^{2+} leaks are shut off near the end of the plateau phase, and Ca^{2+} pumps within the membranes of the sarcoplasmic reticulum and within plasma membranes quickly pump Ca^{2+} out of the intracellular space. This effectively wrests Ca^{2+} away from the contractile mechanism and allows it to relax. Ca^{2+} is thus a major figure in this drama known as excitation–contraction coupling.

SELECTED COMMON ELECTRICAL MALFUNCTIONS

An important impetus for studying cardiac electrophysiology came from the desire to know something about heart disease, and indeed information from the EKGs of patients still continues to contribute to our understanding of normal physiology. Three groups of EKG abnormalities are discussed below to help the reader understand normal function.

Arrhythmias and Conduction Defects

*Conditions That Often Appear in Normal People
and Don't Usually Indicate Disease*

Regular sinus rhythm is the term usually applied when no rhythmic disturbances are seen. It implies that the pacemaker resides in the sinus node and that impulses are generated at regular time intervals.

Sinus tachycardia (Fig. 2.10) on the other hand means that the impulses start properly in the sinus node but occur at a more rapid rate than normal (usually > 100/min). P waves are therefore shaped normally but occur too close together. **Sinus bradycardia** (Fig. 2.11), representing rates < 50/min, describes an unusually slow heart rate at rest. Such slow rates are often seen in athletes, however, and need not imply disease.

Sinus arrhythmia (Fig. 2.12) is often seen in young people and merely means that the heart rate fluctuates in synchrony with respiration. In most subjects the rate increases toward the end of inspiration, but in others it may decrease, and there is no uniform

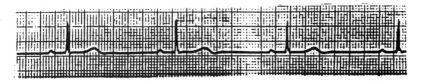
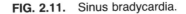

FIG. 2.10. Sinus tachycardia.

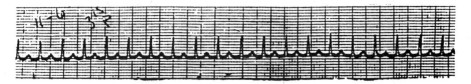

FIG. 2.11. Sinus bradycardia.

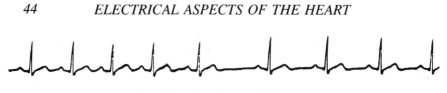

FIG. 2.12. Sinus arrhythmia.

agreement as to its cause. It is likely due to a complex interaction of mechanical and reflex mechanisms.

Another usually benign finding on routine EKGs is the appearance of an occasional **premature ventricular complex** (PVC) (Fig. 2.13). In the usual case the sinus node sends out impulses at a normal rate, but before one such signal can reach the ventricles, a focus within the ventricular mass itself discharges and sends a wave of depolarization throughout the ventricles. Because such a depolarization starts in an unusual locus and is not able to follow the usual His–Purkinje pathway, the QRS pattern for a premature ventricular complex has an aberrant shape and is usually longer in duration than previous normal complexes. The impulse usually does not manage to reach the SA node by traveling retrograde through AV node and atria, and hence the sinus node pacemaker is not reset. Ventricular and possibly AV nodal cells will be in a refractory state following their premature excitation and hence won't respond to the impulse arriving normally from the SA node. The

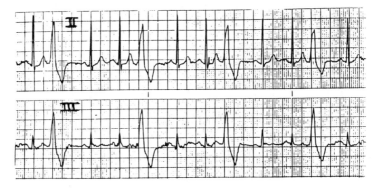

FIG. 2.13. Premature ventricular complex.

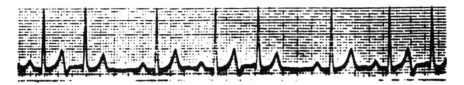

FIG. 2.14.   Premature atrial depolarization.

next sinus impulse will usually find things in order, however, and cause a normal QRS to follow. The result will be a compensatory pause or longer R-R interval immediately following the premature beat. It is even possible to diagnose this condition at the bedside by carefully noting that the premature beat does not disturb the basic cardiac rhythm.

A premature atrial depolarization (Fig. 2.14) is probably no more pathological than its ventricular cousin. The impulse arises outside the sinus node, and the P wave of such a depolarization will usually be shaped differently from an adjacent normal one. Because the sinus node itself gets depolarized, the node will be "reset" and subsequent P waves will be displaced in time.

Conditions That Often Reflect Underlying Cardiac Pathology

In **first-degree AV block** (Fig. 2.15) there is a prolonged delay between the discharge of the sinus node and the corresponding ventricular response. This is reflected in a long P-R interval (time from beginning of the P to beginning of the QRS > 0.2 sec). Because the delay is within or near the AV node, a normal P wave is inscribed.

Second-degree AV block is the general name for a variety of conditions in which AV conduction is interrupted for brief regular

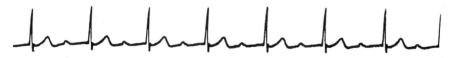

FIG. 2.15.   First-degree AV block.

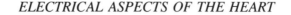

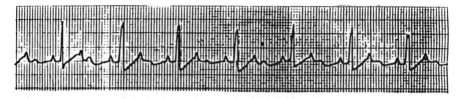

FIG. 2.16.   Second-degree AV block.

periods, but one P wave out of every two, three, or four is still able to traverse the AV node and excite the ventricles. Thus, 2:1 AV block (Fig. 2.16) describes the situation in which only every other P wave is able to reach the ventricles, and there are twice as many P waves as QRS complexes. Such a second-degree block may often occur in association with abnormally high atrial rates and does not necessarily represent pathology within the AV node itself. Note that this gating of too rapid atrial impulses would allow the ventricles to beat at slower, more physiological rates.

A variety of pathologic processes can interrupt impulse propagation down either the left or right bundles, producing **right or left bundle branch block** (Fig. 2.17). When the impulse down one

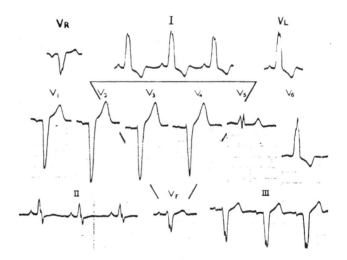

FIG. 2.17.   Left bundle branch block.

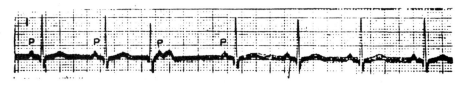

FIG. 2.18.   AV nodal complex.

such bundle is blocked, activation of the ventricle served by that bundle must come via slow transmission from the opposite ventricle. This results in a QRS wider than normal (> 0.12 sec) and a terminal QRS dipole vector pointing toward the offending side. Hence, in right bundle branch block, right ventricular activation will be delayed, and late electrical dipoles will be directed upward toward the right and anteriorly (S waves in leads I, II, and III, and large R$'$ in leads V$_1$ and V$_2$). A right axis deviation of the mean QRS electrical dipole ($> 110°$) will also be present. In left bundle branch block a septal Q wave will be absent, and the late portion of the QRS will be directed upward toward the left and posteriorly.

Premature beats may also originate within the AV node producing an **AV nodal complex** (Fig. 2.18) in which case the usual nodal delay is bypassed, and atria and ventricles are depolarized simultaneously. An upside down P wave is often produced and is usually hidden by the normally appearing QRS.

A common abnormality of the atria, often appearing with no other known pathology, is **paroxysmal atrial tachycardia** (Fig. 2.19). As the name implies the rhythm is abrupt in onset and

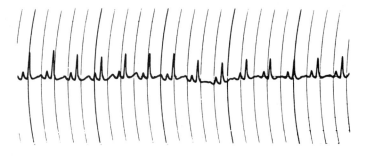

FIG. 2.19.   Paroxysmal atrial tachycardia (dog).

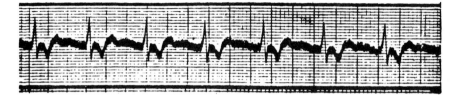

FIG. 2.20.   AV nodal tachycardia.

ending, originates within the atria, and is rapid. Attacks can often be stopped by a Valsalva maneuver (an attempted forced expiration against a closed glottis), carotid sinus massage, or other procedures producing increased vagal discharge. **AV nodal tachycardia** (Fig. 2.20) is usually of a more serious nature and is more difficult to terminate. The absence of discernible P waves is a characteristic feature.

Abnormalities Associated with Serious Underlying Heart Disease

Atrial fibrillation (Fig. 2.21) commonly occurs late in the course of rheumatic heart disease or following myocardial infarction. No normal P waves are seen, but a "wiggly" baseline is often present, representing chaotic waves continually traversing the atria. The AV node prevents most of these from reaching the ventricles, but the impulses that are able to pass through to the ventricles do so at irregular intervals. The QRS response, and therefore the heart rate, is very irregular and often inappropriately rapid.

Atrial flutter (Fig. 2.22) is a more coherent atrial tachycardia, usually associated with a seond-degree 3:1 or 4:1 AV block. The

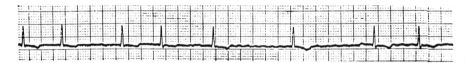

FIG. 2.21.   Atrial fibrillation.

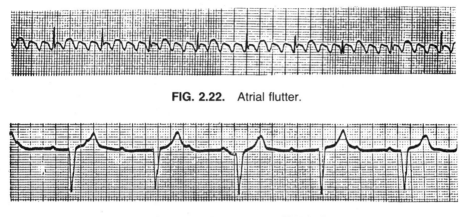

FIG. 2.22. Atrial flutter.

FIG. 2.23. Third-degree AV block.

EKG shows rapid "f" or flutter waves, with only every third or fourth wave eliciting a ventricular QRS response.

Third-degree AV block (Fig. 2.23) is characterized by completely independent rhythms in the atria and ventricles. The former respond to physiologic rate stimuli but the latter beat at an inappropriately slow (30–40/min) idioventricular rate. A permanent third-degree block usually calls for the insertion of an artificial pacemaker with electrodes stimulating the ventricles at a fixed, more rapid rate, or the use of a demand pacemaker which senses the P waves and stimulates the ventricles to respond to each one.

Ventricular tachycardia (Fig. 2.24) is far more serious than its atrial analog and often heralds disaster for the patient. Serious

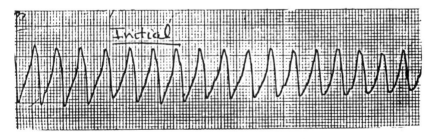

FIG. 2.24. Ventricular tachycardia.

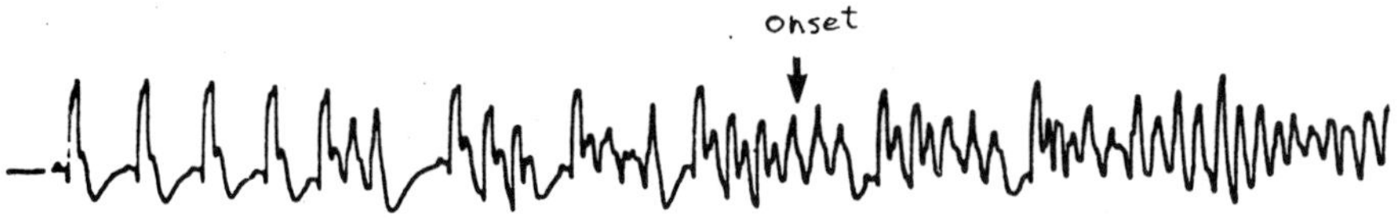

onset

FIG. 2.25. Ventricular fibrillation (dog).

ventricular disease must be present to cause these rapid runs of widened QRS impulses.

Ventricular fibrillation (Fig. 2.25) is incompatible with maintaining life, since the ventricles are not receiving coherent contraction signals. Depolarizing the entire heart with external electrodes (cardioversion) sometimes breaks this pattern and allows the normal mechanism to take over. Often, however, the underlying disease will immediately cause the arrhythmia to recur, and the patient dies.

Ventricular Hypertrophy

In some heart diseases the left or right ventricle hypertrophies, that is, becomes thicker and more massive. For reasons that are not entirely clear, this is associated with larger electrical dipoles in the hypertrophied ventricle, and in later stages with changes in both ST segments and T waves. Severe left ventricular hypertrophy (Fig. 2.26) produces larger than normal dipoles pointing to the

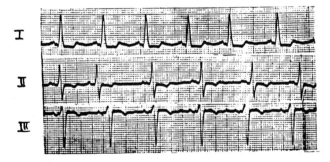

FIG. 2.26. Left ventricular hypertrophy.

left and posteriorly. This will usually be reflected in larger R waves in leads I, V_5, and V_6, and deeper S waves in III, V_1, and V_2. Long-standing disease may produce ST-segment depression and T inversion in I, V_5, and V_6.

Similarly, **right ventricular hypertrophy** allows the normally thinner right heart chamber to assert itself, resulting in larger R waves in the right anterior fields (V_1 and V_2) and in III. As a consequence, the mean electrical axis of the heart is shifted to the right (often past $+110°$) and anteriorly.

Myocardial Infarction

A detailed discussion of **left ventricular infarction** is inappropriate for the beginning physiology student, but several features of this condition should help us in understanding normal physiology. After a sufficiently large coronary artery occlusion, a portion of the heart muscle may die and be replaced by electrically inactive scar tissue. This destroys the dipoles that once were generated in this area: Chest electrodes overlying the region thus show large Q waves and diminished or absent R waves. This is caused by the removal of dipoles that once pointed toward the exploring electrodes and the persistence of dipoles elsewhere in the heart pointing away from the electrodes. During the evolution of an infarct, dying tissue and sick cells adjacent to it are slower to repolarize than they were in health, and, indeed, some of the cell membranes facing the affected area may not be able to repolarize at all. These events often become manifest as inverted T waves or shifted ST segments. (Actually the ST segment stays the same and the rest of the EKG recording shifts, but capacitive coupling in the EKG machine disguises this fact.) Infarcts can also damage various parts of the conduction system, and thereby divert the excitation wave from its normal path. This will show up as late excitation of that part of the ventricle normally served by injured conduction tissue. The pathology can range from a block of the AV node to destruction of some of the finer branches of the Purkinje system.

SUMMARY

Electrical activity in the heart precedes and causes mechanical contraction, and can be recorded as millivolt changes in electrical potential at the body surface. By making arbitrary assumptions regarding (1) normal excitation pathways and (2) a simple dipolar representation of electrical activity, we can sidestep Helmholtz's objections and use these surface potentials to draw conclusions about electrical changes in the heart itself.

QUESTIONS

2.01. Of the four electrical events labeled in the EKG in Fig. 2.27, 1, 2, and 4 are normal for this animal. Event 3 could best be described as a:

a. Premature ventricular complex.   d. Pacemaker prepotential.
b. Premature atrial complex.   e. Electromyogram.
c. Nodal ectopic complex.

2.02. Which one of the six measurements below could not have been recorded from the patient at the same instant as the other five?

a. Lead I = 0.0 mV.   d. Lead aVR = −0.5 mV.
b. Lead II = +1.0 mV.   e. Lead aVL = +0.5 mV.
c. Lead III = +1.0 mV.   f. Lead aVF = +1.0 mV.

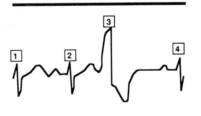

FIG. 2.27.   See Question 2.01.

2.03. Lead II from an elderly man shows P-P intervals that are regularly 0.85 sec while the R-R intervals are regularly 1.9 sec. The most likely diagnosis is:

a. Sinus arrhythmia.
b. Incomplete right bundle branch block.
c. Second-degree heart block.
d. Idioventricular rhythm.
e. Excessive activity of the cardiac sympathetic nerves.

The record in Fig. 2.28 was obtained from an anesthetized dog. It shows the aortic blood pressure and the lead II EKG before and after right vagal stimulation was begun. The stimulation, once begun at the arrow, continued during the rest of the record. Use this record for solving **Questions 2.04 and 2.05.**

2.04. The record shows conclusively the existence of:

a. First-degree AV block.   d. Nodal rhythm.
b. Second-degree AV block.   e. Atrial fibrillation.
c. Third-degree AV block.

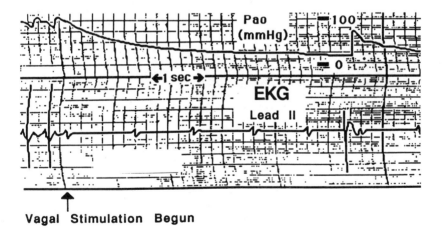

Vagal Stimulation Begun

FIG. 2.28. See Questions 2.04 and 2.05.

2.05. The major reason the arterial pressure fell during the record was:

   a. Ventricular asystole.
   b. Atrial asystole.
   c. Increased arterial compliance.
   d. Decreased arteriolar resistance.
   e. Decreased venous tone.

2.06. What might be the effect of raising the transmembrane potential of (hyperpolarizing) the pacemaker cells?

2.07. If g_K slowly decreased, what would happen to a cell's resting membrane potential?

2.08. How could acetylcholine administration lower ventricular rates via its effect on the AV node?

2.09. What changes in QRS shape would you expect to find associated with isolated AV nodal premature complexes?

ANSWERS

2.01. a. It has all earmarks of a premature ventricular complex, including: (1) QRS is bizarre; (2) QRS is prolonged; (3) T wave is opposite in direction to main part of QRS; (4) QRS merges into T wave without return to isoelectric line; (5) QRS is not necessarily preceded by P wave; and (6) "compensatory pause" is seen.

2.02. e. Use an Einthoven triangle or hexaxial coordinates. Leads I, II, III, aVR, and aVF are consistent with a frontal plane vector pointing vertically down. Lead aVL is not.

2.03. d. There is no consistent relationship between the P waves and the QRS complexes, and the latter are occurring very infrequently (about 32/min). Ventricular pacemakers tend to have rates in the neighborhood of 30–35/min.

2.04. c. The P waves without QRS complexes following the onset of vagal stimulation define third-degree AV block.

2.05. a. If the ventricle puts no blood into the arterial reservoir while blood continues to leak from that reservoir to the tissues, the pressure decreases.

2.06. If one hyperpolarized the pacemaker cells, the prepotential would take longer to decay to the threshold, and thus the heart rate must decrease.

2.07. A cell's resting membrane potential (-70 to -90 mV) is dominated by a high potassium conductance (g_K). This conductance drives the membrane potential toward the potassium equilibrium potential, which tends to be between -90 and -100 mV. If this conductance were to decrease, the cell's resting membrane potential would move towards 0 mV (in a depolarizing direction).

2.08. It could cause a second-degree AV block.

2.09. None. The pathway of ventricular depolarization and thus the QRS would be normal.

3

Physics of the Heart and Circulation

INTRODUCTION

This section presents the circulatory variables: volume, flow, pressure, resistance, compliance, and wall stress, and shows how some of these are measured. Using these variables, the response of the circulatory system to changing external conditions in the absence of controls such as nerves and hormones is explored. Don't let all the quantitation involved throw you. Although the physics is quite necessary in dealing with quantifiable phenomena, the approach is kept as simple as possible. After reading this material you should be able to predict, for example, what would happen to the arterial pressure wave when arteries become stiffer or when arteriolar resistance is increased. You should also be able to predict the effect of ventricular enlargement on afterload. In these and other similar cases you should be able to give quantitative answers.

VOLUMES OF DILUTION

The volume of dilution principle is contained within the definition of concentration:

$$\text{Concentration} = \text{amount/volume} \qquad [3.1]$$

or,

$$\text{Volume} = \text{amount/concentration}$$

Thus, if we could inject a known amount of dye or other marker substance into a fluid within a container and mix it perfectly, we could calculate the volume of the fluid as the amount of dye injected divided by the mixed concentration. This general principle is used to measure volumes of fluid within the body, such as the extracellular space or the circulating blood volume, as well as volumes of gases within the lung. It is necessary to know how much of the injected marker still remains in the system when you measure the concentration. This means taking into account losses that might have occurred, such as in the urinary excretion of extracellular fluid markers or the capillary leakage of plasma volume markers. You also have to be careful in your choice of a marker: You wouldn't use sucrose to mark the plasma volume because it equilibrates with all the water in the extracellular space. So use it to measure the extracellular space. The blue dye T1824, on the other hand, would be good for measuring plasma volume because it sticks to plasma proteins which only very slowly move into the extracellular space.

The requirement for rapid mixing of the marker with the measured volume is self-evident but is pushed to the limit when we attempt to measure the volume of a cardiac chamber, such as the left ventricular cavity, by rapidly injecting a dye into it at some part of the cardiac cycle. If thorough mixing doesn't occur in this circumstance, then downstream at the arterial sampling site there could be inappropriately high or low concentrations depending on which part of the incompletely mixed volume was flowing by at the time of sampling.

Consider some of the markers used in physiological studies:

Plasma volume can be estimated by mixing the protein binding blue dye T1824 into the circulation. Some leakage into the extravascular space will occur, and in order to get a proper measure of concentration, one often extrapolates the concentration versus time curve backward in time to get the concentration at zero time (the time of injection). ^{51}Cr may be used to measure total body red cell volume in much the same way by injecting ^{51}Cr-labeled red cells and measuring their final concentration in radioactivity per volume of cells after mixing. Knowing the radioactivity per volume of blood sampled (not just per red cell volume) will enable one to calculate the circulating blood volume in the same experiment.

Consider an example: ^{51}Cr was complexed to a sample of red cells taken from a patient, and an aliquot containing 55,000 dpm (disintegrations per minute) was reinjected into the patient. After allowing for thorough mixing of the labeled red cells, a 10-ml sample of blood withdrawn from the subject was found to contain 100 dpm of radioactivity. Substitution in Eq. 3.1 yields 5,500 ml as the circulating blood volume. An important assumption is that no radioactivity was lost from the vascular compartment between the times of injection and sampling.

Total body water can be measured using tritiated water, $(^{3}H)_2O$, with sampling from the plasma compartment to get the relevant concentration. The assumption common to that in many such measurements is that the concentration of tritiated water in plasma is the same as that in all body compartments.

^{24}Na may be used to estimate what is called the sodium space by injecting into and sampling from the plasma as above, and then plugging into Eq. 3.1. The result will not be a physically identifiable volume because ^{24}Na concentration is much lower in cells than in extracellular space. Other electrolytes such as ^{42}K and ^{45}Ca are used in a similar fashion in experimental studies.

Lung gas volumes can be estimated at different points in the respiratory cycle using nonradioactive gases such as helium and measuring their concentrations after rebreathing in a closed system. It is essential in such a measurement that no significant loss of marker gas occurs into the bloodstream from the airspaces, or that such losses, if they occur, are accounted for.

The special case of a very rapidly excreted marker is interesting. The marker is cold blood and the volume measured is that of the right ventricular cavity. A catheter is used to inject the blood directly into the ventricle, and samples are taken from an artery downstream. Concentration in this case is the temperature difference between the cooled blood in a sample and the normal warm blood found elsewhere in the subject. Heat exchange is so rapid in capillary beds downstream from the sampling site that no cooled blood recircu-

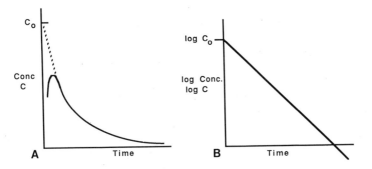

FIG. 3.1.   Idealized curves of concentration versus time.

lates again through the heart. Such recirculation is ordinarily a
serious problem when using dyes for a measurement. Figure 3.1
shows two idealized plots of concentration versus time that might
be found in this case. Because the washout of a ventricular chamber
if often an exponential process, a plot of log concentration versus
time is usually linear. This enables us to extrapolate the concentration
back to the time of injection where we know precisely the amount
of marker within the ventricle. Dividing amount by concentration
gives us the ventricular volume, providing that mixing was rapid
and adequate following injection.

FLOW

Dye Curves

Cardiac output (the flow out of one of the ventricles) can also
be determined from data like those in Fig. 3.1. Practical curves
are seldom as idealized as in that figure, and the data usually look
more like that in Fig. 3.2. We need a little physics here to derive
our formula. The underlying assumption is that the amount of marker
(dI) passing a sampling site in a short time interval (dt) will be
given by the product of the instantaneous concentration (C), the
flow ($\dot{Q}$), and the time interval (dt):

$$dI = \dot{Q} \; C \; dt \qquad\qquad [3.2]$$

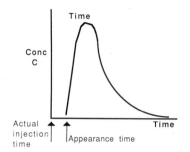

FIG. 3.2. Practical curves of concentration versus time.

The amount of marker passing in infinite time just downstream from a ventricle is given by the integral of Eq. 3.2, and this is also equal to the amount injected (I_0):

$$I_0 = \dot{Q} \, C \, dt \qquad [3.3]$$

In all such examples one assumes a steady state in which flow is constant during the period of measurement. This allows us to take $\dot{Q}$ out from under the integral sign and solve for it:

$$\dot{Q} = I_0/C \, dt \qquad [3.4]$$

This is handy because the denominator of the equation is the area under the concentration/time curve (Fig. 3.2). If we have such a plot of concentration versus time, we can obtain a graphical estimate of this integral and can calculate a flow without having to know the actual function that describes how concentration varies with time.

Most dyes will recirculate through the vascular bed, however, artificially raising the concentration as they revisit the sampling site. This means that dye curves will look something like Fig. 3.3a, in which the area under the curve will be infinite if taken to infinite time. An arbitrary way to get around this is to plot the natural log (ln) of concentration as in Fig. 3.3b. One then assumes that the real concentration versus time curve would have an exponential shape in the absence of recirculation, and focuses on the usually short linear portion of the ln concentration/time curve just prior to

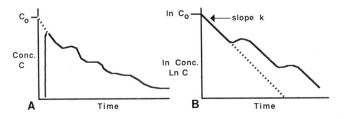

FIG. 3.3. Dye curves: showing recirculation. **a:** Concentration versus time. **b:** Ln concentration versus time.

the recirculation hump. We start this time with Eq. 3.4, which still holds, but note that the logarithmic process

$$\ln C = \ln C_0 + kt \qquad [3.5]$$

can also be expressed in exponential terms:

$$C = C_0 e^{kt} \qquad [3.6a]$$

Here C is the instantaneous concentration, C_0 is its value at $t = 0$, and k is the slope of the linear portion of the curve on the natural logarithmic plot. In any real system k will have a negative value, given by:

$$k = \ln(C_2/C_1)/(t_2 - t_1) \qquad [3.6b]$$

We can then get the area under the concentration/time curve (Fig. 3.2) by integrating Eq. 3.6a from zero to infinite time:

$$C_0 e^{kt} \, dt = -C_0/k \qquad [3.7]$$

which can be substituted into Eq. 3.4 to give:

$$\dot{Q} = -kI_0/C_0 \qquad [3.8]$$

C_0 is obtained by graphic extrapolation to $t = 0$. Because k is always negative, $\dot{Q}$ is always positive. It is important to remember that Eq. 3.8 embodies the assumption that washout of a chamber is an exponential process.

Because natural (base e) semilog paper is hard to find, we could plot the data on ordinary (base 10) semilog paper, calculate a slope,

$k' = \log(C_2/C_1)/(t_2 - t_1)$, and then let $k = 2.303k'$. This adjusts for the use of base 10 logs in an inherently natural or base e situation. The usual procedure is to plot the data on base 10 semilog paper and calculate k directly from the printed values of C on the ordinate, because ordinate values have already been converted from logarithmic to linear form. One can merely plug these numbers into the definition above: $k = \ln(C_2/C_1)/(t_2 - t_1)$. Bear in mind that k is the true slope of the natural semilog plot, **not** the slope of the base 10 semilog plot.

If all this seems terribly difficult to remember, we suggest that you merely memorize Eq. 3.8 and the definitions of k and C_0.

Fick Principle

A more traditional approach to the determination of cardiac output involves the Fick principle, illustrated in Fig. 3.4. The conservation principles underlying the Fick relationship are also used to derive most of the other equations employed in respiratory and renal physiology. The Fick equation is easily derived by making use of the steady-state assumption that the flow of O_2 into the lung is equal to the flow of O_2 out. The O_2 input has two components: (1) net O_2 input into the lung via the airway, known as $\dot{V}O_2$ (remember that the exhaled air carries a lot of O_2), and (2) O_2 carried by the blood flow, $\dot{Q}$, in the pulmonary artery. The latter is largely bound to hemoglobin, but some is in solution in the plasma and cell water; we shall call the total concentration $C_{PA}O_2$. Input via the bloodstream is thus $\dot{Q} \times C_{PA}O_2$. The pulmonary veins conduct

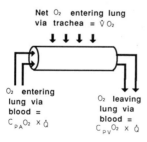

FIG. 3.4.   Fick principle: O_2 flow in = O_2 flow out.

the only net flow of O_2 out of the lung, and this is given as $\dot{Q} \times C_{PV}O_2$.

Making the steady-state assumptions that both O_2 flow and blood flow are constant, we can equate O_2 input with output:

$$\dot{Q} \times C_{PA}O_2 + \dot{V}O_2 = \dot{Q} \times C_{PV}O_2 \qquad [3.9]$$

Rearranging this gives us the Fick equation, Eq. 3.10, which is as useful in the cardiac catheterization lab as it is on physiology tests. Please memorize it.

$$\dot{Q} = \frac{\dot{V}O_2}{C_{PV}O_2 - C_{PA}O_2} \qquad [3.10]$$

The same equation can be used to calculate blood flow through any other organ. One needs to know only the concentrations of O_2 in the blood entering and leaving the organ, and the net uptake of O_2 by the organ. The principle is of course not limited to O_2, and can be applied to CO_2 and other substrates as well if the necessary concentrations and uptake are known.

It is important to realize that the Fick equation **can be applied only within a region of the circulation where we have:**

1. a flow of blood into the region and a measured concentration of a substance in that blood;
2. a source or sink for that substance **within the region** and a measurement of the appearance or disappearance rate of that substance; and
3. the same flow of blood out of the region and a measured concentration of the same substance in that blood.

One could use the equation to calculate muscle blood flow if one knew, say, the concentration of CO_2 in arterial blood entering the region, the time rate of production of CO_2 by that muscle, and the concentration of CO_2 in venous blood draining that muscle. One could **not** use the equation with O_2 concentrations to calculate directly the flow of blood through the ventricle, because there is no measureable source or sink for O_2 within the left ventricle.

Try a calculation. What is the cardiac output in a man at rest if his pulmonary venous O_2 content is 200 ml O_2/L blood, his pulmonary arterial O_2 content is 150 ml O_2/L blood and his body O_2 uptake is 250 ml O_2/min? Answer: (250 ml O_2/min)/[(200 − 150) ml O_2/L blood] = 5 L blood/min.

Here's a harder one. What are the pulmonary, systemic, and shunt blood flows in a patient with an interventricular septal defect and a left to right shunt, given that:

$$C_{PA O_2} = 180,$$
$$C_{PV O_2} = 200,$$
$$C_{AO O_2} = 200, \text{ and}$$
$$C_{RA O_2} = 150 \text{ ml } O_2/\text{L blood, and}$$
$$\dot{V}_{O_2} = 250 \text{ ml } O_2/\text{min.}$$

The situation is pictured in Fig. 3.5. To solve the problem, first calculate the pulmonary blood flow as 250/(200 − 180) = 12.5 L/min, and then the systemic flow as 250/(200 − 150) = 5 L/min. The shunt flow must be the difference between the two or 7.5 L/min from the left ventricle to the right, across the septum. It is common in severe cases of this congenital deformity for the left heart to be putting more blood through the defect than through the aorta. To get a solution, one must realize that in the steady state $\dot{V}_{O_2}$ represents net O_2 flow into the lungs as well as into the tissues.

In applying this method clinically, one must be careful to achieve a steady state and truly representative blood samples. Brachial or

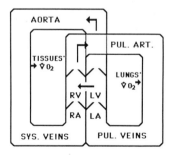

FIG. 3.5. Interventricular septal defect. LA, left atrium; LV, left ventricle; RA, right atrium; RV, right ventricle.

femoral arterial samples are often used to estimate pulmonary venous O_2 contents and will be strongly affected by right to left shunts. Small shunts of this kind occur normally through the Thebesian veins draining into the left ventricular cavity and via the bronchial circulation.

PRESSURE

Transmural Pressures and Driving Pressures

Pressures in the body are always measured as **differences** from some reference level. Often the reference level is ambient atmospheric pressure, because most pressure gauges have one side open to room air. Therefore, the average blood pressure in large arteries is often found to be 95 mm Hg, meaning 95 mm Hg above atmospheric pressure. At the same time, the average **transmural** (across the wall) pressure in these same arteries might be 90 mm Hg. This means that intraarterial pressure minus periarterial tissue pressure is approximately 95 − 5 or 90 mm Hg. The convention in using transmural pressures is to take inside minus outside pressure. Arterial pressure is also involved in the **driving** pressure of approximately 95 mm Hg, which drives blood through the systemic vascular resistance. Measurements here are required from both ends of the vascular beds involved, with the result again being expressed as a difference, in this case 95 mm Hg (aorta) minus 0 mm Hg (right atrium). Figure 3.6 summarizes these relationships.

Methods of Pressure Measurement

Although volume and flow are difficult to measure, vascular pressures are relatively easy to determine, even at the bedside.

Perhaps the simplest and most direct such measurement involves the determination of a patient's venous pressure by observing his neck veins. Figure 3.7 illustrates how the height to which the column of blood rises in these veins is identical to the height of the fluid column in a saline-filled manometer. The reference point in each

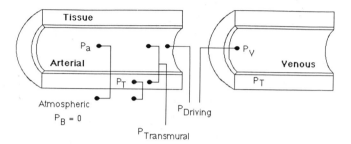

Arterial Pressure	=	$P_a - P_B$
Tissue Pressure	=	$P_T - P_B$
Transmural Arterial Pressure	=	$P_a - P_T$
Transmural Venous Pressure	=	$P_V - P_T$
Systemic Driving Pressure	=	$P_a - P_V$

FIG. 3.6. Pressures.

of these cases is usually taken as the level of the right atrium (where venous pressure is **normally** close to atmospheric pressure, defined as zero). Thus, the height of a blood column or manometer meniscus above the right atrium reports elevations of pressure within that structure. Such venous pressures are often reported in units of centimeters of water (cm H_2O). An open manometer indicates pressure as the height to which its fluid is pushed against gravity

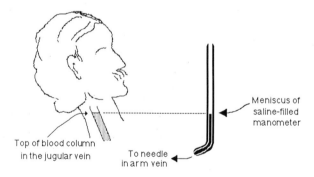

FIG. 3.7. Jugular venous manometer.

by the pressure. The height of the column of fluid is often taken directly as the reading, although it can be translated into more austere units by calculating:

$$p = \rho g h \qquad [3.11]$$

where ρ is the specific gravity of the fluid, g is the acceleration due to gravity, and h is the height of the fluid column. Using mercury as a fluid, ρ is 13.6×10^3 kg/m^3 and g is 9.80 m/sec^2, average arterial blood pressure will support a mercury column of 93 mm (0.093 m) against gravity and atmospheric pressure, hence

$$P = (13.6 \times 10^3)(9.80)(0.093) = 12{,}400 \text{ Newtons/m}^2$$
$$= 12.4 \text{ kilo Pascals}$$

Neither Newton nor Pascal was aware of this.

Arterial pressure measurement requires a bit of explanation. One uses a sphygmomanometer, but calls it a blood pressure cuff (Fig. 3.8). The cuff is placed around the subject's upper arm and inflated to a reading well above the expected systolic pressure. By listening with a stethoscope over the brachial artery in the antecubital fossa just below the cuff and slowly releasing cuff pressure, the observer can hear the first squirts of blood that are allowed to pass through the squeezed artery. The cuff pressure reading at this point is very close to the systolic or highest phasic pressure in the artery. As the cuff continues to deflate, the sounds will change abruptly in quality or disappear altogether, marking the diastolic or lowest phasic pressure in the artery.

The sounds are called Korotkoff sounds, after their discoverer, and are produced only when blood is flowing **intermittently** in the compressed artery. They are apparently associated with rapid acceleration and deceleration of the blood flow as arterial pressure exceeds and then falls below the external cuff pressure. When cuff pressure is above systolic as in A in Fig. 3.8b, there is no flow and no sound. When cuff pressure is at some point below systolic but above diastolic, flow must start and stop at pressure B in the figure. At pressures below diastolic, for example C in Fig. 3.8b, flow is smooth and continuous and no sound is produced.

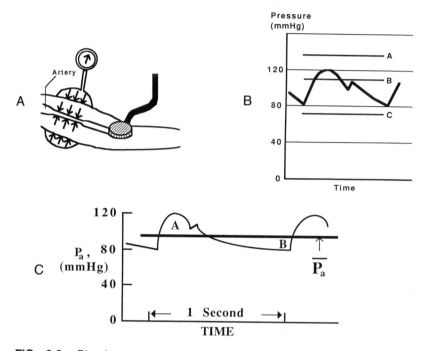

FIG. 3.8. Blood pressure measurement. **a:** Sphygmomanometer and stethoscope. **b:** Arterial pressure wave. **c:** Determination of mean arterial pressure.

During diagnostic heart catheterization, long flexible tubes are inserted via arteries and veins into the innermost recesses of the right and left heart and the lung. Pressures are usually monitored continuously with electrical strain gauge pressure transducers which can record arterial, ventricular, and other pulse waves. Even higher fidelity recordings can be made with a pressure sensor placed on the catheter tip.

Effects of Gravity, Posture, and Surrounding Pressure

Pressures in the cardiovascular system are very sensitive to body position, although normal right and left atrial pressures are always close to atmospheric pressure. Therefore, venous pressure in your big toe rises on quiet standing because of the long uninterrupted column of venous blood connecting it to the right atrium. Working against such high venous pressures might seem very difficult. Fortunately, however, arteries must obey the same physical laws as veins, and arterial pressures in the big toe are correspondingly high because the artery to the big toe also sits beneath its own column of blood connected to the heart.

A somewhat different but related problem is experienced at the other end of the body. Because the brain is located some tens of centimeters above the heart, brain venous pressure is subatmospheric. The situation is complicated by the neck veins, which tend to collapse when outside pressure exceeds inside pressure, as in this case. Pressure within such veins is close to atmospheric throughout their course. Venous pressure within the skull, however, is still slightly subatmospheric, and these veins are prevented from collapsing by the skull surrounding them. Be careful, the insertion of needles into veins above the heart can allow air to be sucked into the vascular system.

Venous pressures in your legs can rise precipitously when you stand up suddenly. The dizziness you experience on such occasions results from blood pooling in your distended leg veins instead of perfusing your head adequately. Your body comes to your rescue, however. By increasing venous tone (increased active tension or stress in the muscles within vein walls), it delivers blood to the heart for redistribution to more deserving organs.

The vessels and heart chambers lying within the chest cavity are subject to increasingly negative pressures during inspiration and less negative pressures during expiration. This serves to pull blood into the chest during inspiration and to expel it during expiration. This "thoracic pump" aids cardiac output, particularly during exercise when intrathoracic pressure swings are greatest.

Shape of the Arterial Pressure Wave

The arterial pressure wave has a curious shape (Fig. 3.8b), with a bump on its downswing following what is called the dicrotic notch. The notch occurs at the same time as closure of the aortic valve and perhaps represents a bouncing wave due to this event.

The pulse wave in the leg differs from those closer to the heart by being somewhat skinnier and taller. Mean leg arterial pressure is slightly lower than more centrally measured pressures, but selective, more rapid transmission of high-frequency pressure-wave components down the arteries results in leg systolic pressures being higher than arm systolic pressures. When leg systolic pressures are lower than arm systolic pressures, look for a possible obstructive aortic lesion such as a coarctation of the aorta or perhaps severe arteriosclerosis.

Mean arterial pressure in the arms is not usually the average of systolic and diastolic pressures. Fig. 3.8c illustrates how to determine the mean arterial pressure, which is the constant pressure whose blood driving ability is the same as the fluctuating pressure actually found in the arteries. It must be chosen so that the pressure–time area under the pulse wave and over the constant pressure line (area A) is equal to the pressure–time area over the pulse wave and under the constant pressure line (area B). The location of this constant pressure line is usually determined electronically.

The mean brachial arterial pressure can be estimated fairly accurately in a resting person whose heart rate and pulse wave contours are normal, however, by using a weighted average involving two parts diastolic and one part systolic pressure. Thus, mean Pa $\sim$ $(P_{sys} + 2(P_{dias})/3$, and the typical person at rest will therefore have a mean arterial pressure of about 93 mm Hg.

RESISTANCE

Definition

Circulatory resistance is usually defined as the driving pressure divided by the concomitant flow. It's like Ohm's law for electricity in which resistance is equal to voltage drop divided by current flow: $R = E/I$. It's just as well you memorize:

$$P_1 - P_2 = P_{driving} = R \times \dot{Q} \qquad [3.12]$$

The components are illustrated in Fig. 3.9.

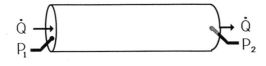

FIG. 3.9. Driving pressure.

Poiseuille–Hagen Law

The science of hydraulics was fostered and the lives of physiology students were complicated by the discovery in the last century that the flow of most fluids through tubes was proportional to the fourth power of the radius of the tube, and inversely proportional to the viscosity of the fluid and the length of the tube. Putting together the findings of the physician Poiseuille and the engineer Hagen we can write:

$$P_{\text{driving}} = \frac{8\eta L}{\pi r^4} Q \qquad [3.13]$$

where η represents fluid viscosity, L, the length and r, the radius of the tube, and $\dot{Q}$, the flow through the tube. By comparing Eq. 3.13 with 3.12 one can see that the product of the factors multiplying $\dot{Q}$ is the resistance. Merely doubling the radius will therefore divide resistance by 16 and multiply flow by the same factor. The muscles in arteriolar walls use this relation to advantage in diverting flow from organ to organ within the body.

The viscosity term in Eq. 3.13 becomes important when the red cells become too numerous in blood. The viscosity of plasma, devoid of cells, is approximately 1.8 times that of water. (The viscosity of water is 0.01 poises, or 1 centipoise at 21°C.) Normal blood with a hematocrit of 45% (percent of the blood consisting of cells) has a relative viscosity of 3 to 4 when measured in a viscometer; it can double or triple at higher, sick hematocrits. One might naturally think that this thickening of the blood would require doubling or tripling of arterial pressures to produce the needed blood flow, but two effects in the circulation make such a pressure rise unnecessary. First, blood flow through narrow arterioles and capillaries isn't impeded to the extent that one would predict from viscometer measurements. The ordered, axial streaming of red blood cells through a set of narrow parallel tubes offers a lower resistance to flow than does the less ordered pattern of flow through the larger tubes used in many viscometers. Second, the slightly higher driving pressures required by higher viscosities result in higher transmural pressures across the distensible walls of the resistance vessels, causing them to become more expanded and to offer less resistance to flow than they would have otherwise. The pressure required to perfuse tissues with blood at a hematocrit of 45% is therefore only 10% higher than would be required for plasma alone. The effect of higher hematocrits on vascular resistance thus cannot be calculated from *in vitro* viscosity measurements alone.

Resistances in Series and Parallel

Add two identical pipes together end to end, and the resistance of the ensemble is double that of each piece alone. The same is true of vascular segments, and we can generalize this by saying that resistances in series add directly:

$$R_{T,series} = R_1 + R_2 \qquad [3.14]$$

Put the same pipes side by side instead, and the same driving pressure will obviously get you twice the flow. More generally, we say that resistances in parallel add reciprocally:

$$1/R_{T,parallel} = 1/R_1 + 1/R_2 \qquad [3.15]$$

While numerical resistance calculations aren't commonly used in patient care, they are regularly performed in the cardiac catheterization lab, and they're useful in explaining physiological control mechanisms. Consider, for example, the resistance of the systemic circulation. Taking mean arterial pressure as 93 mm Hg, mean right atrial pressure as 3 mm Hg, and cardiac output as 5 L/min, we can plug into Eq. 3.12 and calculate resistance R to be (93 − 3)/5 = 18 mm Hg/(L/min). The strange units are usually left in this form. High blood pressure (hypertension) is characterized by a significant increase in systemic resistance, which may even double.

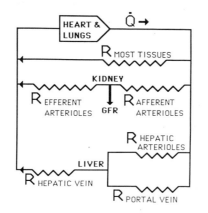

FIG. 3.10.   Series and parallel resistances in the circulation.

Figure 3.10 illustrates the series and parallel nature of our circulation. For example, in cases of shock, kidney blood flow can be markedly decreased by increasing the resistance of the afferent arterioles. On the other hand, when a higher glomerular filtration rate (GFR) is needed, it can be achieved by separately increasing the efferent and decreasing the afferent arteriolar resistance. Precisely what happens in the liver with its complex series/parallel arranged circulation is not fully understood.

ACTIVE AND PASSIVE WALL STRESS— THE LAW OF LAPLACE

The law of Laplace relates radius, transmural pressure, and wall stress (also known as wall tension) in thin-walled, distensible spheres and cylinders. Our analysis will take into account the thickness of these structures as well. It therefore represents a minor (and approximate) extension of the pure Laplace relationship for thin-walled spheres and cylinders.

The concept of **ventricular wall stress** is important for understanding ventricular function. How can it be calculated?

Consider the ventricle to be cut into two hollow hemispheres (Fig. 3.11). In the plane of the cut, the cardiac chamber of radius, r, has a circular cross-sectional area of πr^2. Suppose we stitch

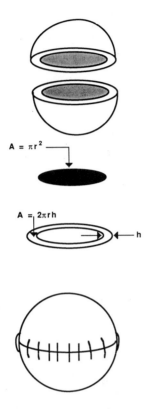

$A = \pi r^2$

$A = 2\pi r h$

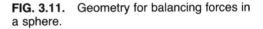

FIG. 3.11. Geometry for balancing forces in a sphere.

the wall back together again all around the chamber, fill it with blood, and set it generating pressure once more. A given transmural pressure, P_{TM}, will act to push the two halves apart with a force, F_{out}, equal to the transmural pressure times the cross-sectional area of the chamber in the slicing plane:

$$F_{out} = P_{TM} \times \pi r^2 \qquad [3.16a]$$

In order for the structure to hold together, the walls must resist this push at the same slicing plane with a force of equal magnitude. This force can be approximated by the product of a pressure or stress within the wall times the wall cross-sectional area in the slicing plane. This wall stress, S_W, is parallel to the wall itself and is perpendicular to the slicing plane. It's like the stitches required to hold the sliced ventricle together. It has the units of pressure, which are force per area. We shall further approximate the wall cross-sectional area by $2\pi rh$, where r is again the radius of the ventricular chamber, and h is the wall thickness. The inward wall force resisting the outward pressure force is therefore given by:

$$F_{in} = S_W \times 2\pi rh \qquad [3.16b]$$

In other words, the total force holding the heart together in this plane is the internal pressure (stress) times the cross-sectional area of the wall itself in this plane. Equating F_{out} and F_{in} yields:

$$P_{TM}\pi r^2 = S_W 2\pi rh \qquad [3.16c]$$

Solving this for wall stress, S_W, gives:

$$S_W = P_{TM}r/(2h) \qquad [3.16d]$$

which is the final form of our (modified) Laplace relationship. If you can't easily derive it, please memorize it.

Equation 3.16d has some important messages for ventricular function, because S_W, wall stress, is probably the most important index of the load on the heart. It is a formula for calculating both the so-called preload and afterload on the heart. You can that wall stress is directly related to transmural pressure (P_{TM}, equivalent to arterial pressure under most circumstances). When wall thickness (h, in the denominator) becomes greater, the stress becomes less, all other factors remaining equal. This is intuitively correct because a thicker ventricle ought to be able to withstand the strain of high pressures more easily. The somewhat surprising feature of Eq. 3.16d is the fact that wall stress is also positively influenced by the size of the ventricle through r, its radius. This means that big ventricles are at an inherent disadvantage (because of larger stress) with respect to normal or small ventricles, even when they are of equal thickness and have to create equal pressures. We want to emphasize here that both the preload (wall stress just before contraction) and afterload (increase of wall stress during contraction) can be estimated by Eq. 3.16d. They will be discussed further in Chapter 4.

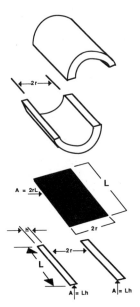

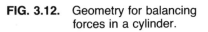

FIG. 3.12.   Geometry for balancing forces in a cylinder.

Vessel wall stress is also an important factor in understanding how the circulation works. It can be estimated by an equation similar to that used in describing ventricular wall stress.

Figure 3.12, analogous to Fig. 3.11, shows the relationships. The total outward force distending a vessel segment of length L and thickness h, directed perpendicular to a slicing plane, is given by the transmural pressure, P_{TM}, times the cross-sectional luminal area in that plane:

$$F_{out} = P_{TM}2rL \qquad [3.17a]$$

The total inward force (perpendicular to the plane) resisting this tendency to expand resides within the vessel wall, and is given by the product of wall stress, S_W, and the cross-sectional area of the wall in the slicing plane:

$$F_{in} = S_W 2Lh \qquad [3.17b]$$

For a stable, nonbursting vessel, these forces must be equal:

$$P_{TM}2rL = S_W 2Lh \qquad [3.17c]$$

and the relationship describing this can be solved for wall stress:

$$S_W = P_{TM}r/h \qquad [3.17d]$$

The resulting Laplace relationship for a thick-walled cylinder differs from that for a thick-walled sphere only by a factor of two. Again, it should be memorized if you can't derive it. Table 3.1 gives very approximate values of wall stresses for three vascular structures. The values are surprisingly similar considering that these vessels vary tremendously in size.

The stress calculated for Table 3.1 actually represents the sum of passive and active stress components in arteries and veins containing contractile muscle units. The interaction of these stresses with radius and transmural pressure in a given structure is often difficult for students to understand, and is discussed in the next section.

Consider Fig. 3.13a which shows the law of Laplace for distensible cylinders in equilibrium states at different constant distending pressures. Each constant pressure line merely shows the state of structures having this fixed, constant transmural pressure. If you decide to work with a fixed distending pressure P_2, then the law of Laplace says that you're stuck on the straight line labeled P_2 no matter what equilibrium cylinder is involved. Such a line implies, for example, that at the same transmural pressure, small cylinders (having small radii) will have smaller stress-times-thickness products than larger cylinders.

Let's momentarily set aside the law of Laplace and consider the behavior of cylindrical blood vessels as they are inflated by

TABLE 3.1 *Wall stresses of different vessels*

Cava	Aorta	Capillary	Vena
$P(N/m^2)$	13330	4000	1333
$r(m)$	13×10^{-3}	4×10^{-6}	16×10^{-3}
$h(m)$	3×10^{-3}	1×10^{-6}	1×10^{-3}
$S_W(N/m^2)$	58×10^3	16×10^3	21×10^3

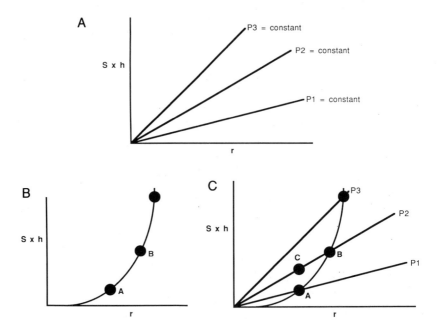

FIG. 3.13. Law of Laplace in a blood vessel. **a:** Laplace's law. **b:** Passive vessel. **c:** Laplace's law and vessel characteristics.

blood or fluid. To see how one particular vessel, a **passive** vein, might actually behave, have a look at Fig. 3.13b. Here we are describing not one particular pressure as in Fig. 13a, but one particular physical structure, in this case a vein. Note that the shape of this curve is characteristic of many anatomic structures: At low radii (low volume) stress times thickness changes relatively less with radius than at higher radii (high volume) where stress times thickness changes a lot with a given change in radius. That is, the walls tend to be stiffer at higher volumes. This is also true for balloons, for example. (This curve might have been constructed by distending the vessel with different pressures (P_1, P_2, and P_3, for example) and then measuring radius, wall thickness, and wall stress.) In the following analysis we shall assume that vessel wall thickness, h, remains essentially constant as the vessel expands.

This is a reasonable approximation for small expansions, but does not apply when radius is more than doubled.

Let's now put Laplace's law and the vessel's characteristics together in Fig. 3.13c. Consider a particular pressure, P_1. The law of Laplace says that the straight line labeled P_1 is the locus of all points for a vessel at equilibrium. The only possible equilibrium state for this particular vein is therefore the intersection of the curve and the straight line, and this is shown as point A in Fig. 3.13c. The law of Laplace will hold for all points on the curve such that S always equals Pr/h, but if we want to stretch the vessel to larger radii, we'll have to use higher pressures, and therefore move to a point (e.g., point B) at the intersection of the curve with a higher pressure line.

Now let's complicate things and see what **could** happen if we **kept transmural pressure constant** and varied r by activating muscles in the vessel wall. The addition of **active** wall stress will make the vessel (and its radius) smaller. Let's start at point B on the passive curve in Fig. 3.13c. We can't get away from Laplace, and because we are keeping pressure constant, we must follow the straight line labeled P_2 in the figure (because $Sh = Pr,$ and P, the slope, is constant). We couldn't have gone to the right of the passive curve, even if we had wanted to, because the vessel was completely relaxed to start with. However, if we make the vessel contract actively, causing its radius to become smaller, we will move down P_2 to the left, off the passive curve and into the active area of the plot. This will take us to point C, where the active stress component is given as the difference in stresses between point C and point A on the **passive** stress line directly below C. The passive component of stress is given by the stress at A.

This is roughly how arterioles and veins work. Muscles in their walls contract, increasing **active** stress and moving blood above and to the left of the old passive stress line. Veins do this to decrease their volume, increase their transmural pressure, and effectively give the rest of the circulation a transfusion. Arterioles do it to increase their resistance (while tending to raise the pressure at the input end but lowering it at the output end).

COMPLIANCE

Compliance (distensibility or stretchability, the opposite of stiffness) is a property of many biological structures. Veins are reasonably flimsy vessels, more compliant than thick-walled arteries of comparable diameter. We quantitate compliance by measuring the **change** in volume produced by a **change** in transmural pressure:

$$C = \Delta V / \Delta P_{TM} \qquad [3.18]$$

The point often difficult to grasp is that we use a **change** or difference in transmural pressure. Transmural pressure itself already represents a difference in pressure between the inside and outside of the structure involved. This difference between differences is summarized in Fig. 3.14. Don't yield to temptation and substitute a mere transmural pressure in this relation. Keep in mind also that in this and most other physiological writing, transmural pressure means inside pressure minus outside pressure. Changes over time are usually measured as final situation minus initial situation.

Compliance is particularly useful in discussing the respiratory system, but it is also relevant to our consideration of the stiffness of heart chambers or vessels. For example, how can you calculate the approximate compliance of the arterial tree, using circulatory data you already know? Consider the stroke volume pushed into the aorta with each beat of the heart. When an average cardiac output of 5 L/min is divided by a resting heart rate of 72, we get a stroke volume of 69 ml. This volume is added to the arterial circulation while the aortic valve is open. Because systole lasts

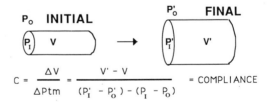

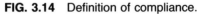

$$C = \frac{\Delta V}{\Delta P tm} = \frac{V' - V}{(P_I' - P_o') - (P_I - P_o)} = \text{COMPLIANCE}$$

FIG. 3.14 Definition of compliance.

for about one-third of the cardiac cycle, however, one-third of this stroke volume will be leaking out of the arteries into the arterioles while the heart is contracting, leaving a net addition of only $(2/3) \times$ 69 or 46 ml as our ΔV.

During the short period of time that this net volume addition to the arteries occurs, arterial pressure goes from its lowest (diastolic) value of approximately 80 mm Hg when the aortic valve opens, to a maximum of 120 mm Hg, and then back down to about 110 mm Hg when the aortic valves close. There is a net increase in pressure of $110 - 80 = 30$ mm Hg over this time period, and this is associated with a net volume increase of 46 ml, giving an arterial compliance of $46/30 = 1.5$ ml/mm Hg.

The stiff arteries of arteriosclerosis are associated with normal stroke volumes and high differences between systolic and diastolic pressures (pulse pressure). Their compliance is often only half that of normal arteries. Mean pressures are commonly not elevated in this situation, merely the systolic pressure. Hence, this is not true hypertension (high blood pressure), which in addition requires that the diastolic and mean pressures also be raised above normal.

We can also estimate the compliance of the human veins-plus-venules reservoir by considering that decreasing its volume by 750 ml would be associated with a decrease in its average transmural pressure from 7 to 0 mm Hg (in the absence of compensatory reflex changes). This gives a venous compliance of $750/(7 - 0)$ $= 110$ ml/mm Hg. So, venous compliance is something like 70 times larger than arterial compliance, or alternatively, our arterial system is roughly 70 times as stiff as our venous system.

Having estimates of these circulatory compliances allows us to consider what would happen in our (very difficult) experiment of starting the circulation from scratch. We'll begin with the situation pictured in Fig. 3.15a, in which $\dot{Q} = 0$, and pressure everywhere in the vasculature is 7 mm Hg (equals the mean circulatory pressure, P_{MC}).

We shall set the systemic vascular resistance to a normal value of about 20 mm Hg/(L/min), 19 units of which are contributed by the arterioles and capillaries, and 1 unit of which is contributed

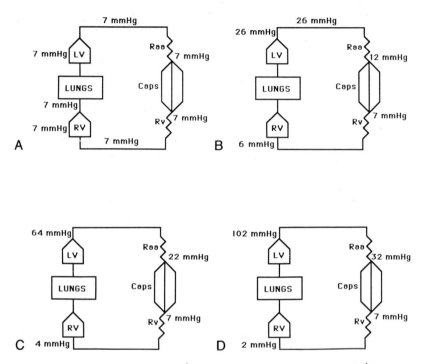

FIG. 3.15. Pressure when **(a)** $\dot{Q} = 3$ L/min (heart stopped); **(b)** $\dot{Q} = 1$ L/min; **(c)** $\dot{Q} = 3$ L/min; and **(d)** $\dot{Q} = 5$ L/min.

by the venules and veins. We shall set the venous/venular compliance to about 60 times that of the arteries.

Figure 3.15b depicts the steady-state situation which might result if the $\dot{Q}$ were raised to 1 L/min and kept there long enough to obtain measurements. Note that the pressure remains 7 mm Hg ($= P_{MC}$) only in the postcapillary venules and changes everywhere else. It becomes greater than 7 mm Hg in the arteries, arterioles, and capillaries, and less than 7 mm Hg in the great veins and the right atrium. The pressure drop from arteries to right atrium is now 20 mm Hg, in keeping with $\dot{Q} = 1$ L/min and the $R_{sys} = 20$ mm Hg/(L/min).

The pressure in the arteries has increased from 7 mm Hg (when

$\dot{Q} = 0$) to 26 mm Hg (now that $\dot{Q} = 1$ L/min), a change of 19 mm Hg. This increase, and the decrease in right atrial and great venous pressures, is due to the transfer of a volume of blood from the venous reservoir to the arterial reservoir. We can use the just-calculated arterial compliance of 1.5 ml/mm Hg and the ΔP_a of 19 mm Hg to estimate that the arterial volume has been increased by almost 30 ml.

It is more difficult to estimate a single value for the change in pressure in the venous reservoir because it involves many different structures lying in the path from the capillaries to the right atrium. A useful approximation of average pressure in the venous reservoir might be: (right atrial pressure + $2P_{MC}$)/3. According to this formula, the average pressure in the venous reservoir has fallen from 7.00 to 6.67 mm Hg. The rise in arterial pressure is so much larger than the fall in venous pressure because the compliance of the arteries is only 1/60 that of the veins.

Fig. 3.15c shows another instantaneous picture of the system with $\dot{Q}$ at 3 L/min. The arterial pressure has increased to 64 mm Hg and the right atrial pressure has fallen to 4 mm Hg while the postcapillary pressure has stayed at the $P_{MC} = 7$ mm Hg. Between the situation pictured in Fig. 3.15a and that in 3.15c, a total of 86 ml has been transferred from veins to arteries. Finally, in Fig. 3.15d, $\dot{Q}$ (5 L/min) and the pressures in the arteries (102 mm Hg) and the right atrium (2 mm Hg) have reached their normal resting values. A total of about 143 ml of blood has been transferred from veins to arteries during the time interval between Figs. 3.15a and 3.15d.

Besides stressing the pressure connection between resistance and compliance, this kind of exercise also points out an important clinical generalization. That is that each step increase of cardiac output in Fig. 3.15 led to an increase in arterial pressure and a decrease in right atrial pressure. The pumping action of the heart serves to keep arterial pressure high and venous pressure low. Whenever a ventricle becomes a better and more effective pump, the pressure in the veins returning blood to that ventricle (and the filling pressure of that ventricle) decreases. Thus, increases in contractility (and to some extent increases in heart rate) and decreases in afterload tend to reduce venous pressure.

In ventricular failure, on the other hand, contractility is lower than normal, resulting in a less effective pump and causing the filling pressure of that ventricle to rise. Right ventricular failure, therefore, causes a rise in systemic venous pressure, which in turn is often associated with increased systemic capillary pressure and peripheral tissue edema. Similarly, left ventricular failure is associated with a rise in pulmonary venous pressure, which can lead to high pulmonary capillary pressures and pulmonary edema. This latter can be life threatening.

From a clinical diagnostic point of view, one should therefore suspect a failing right ventricle when systemic venous pressures rise and a failing left ventricle when pulmonary venous pressures rise.

HEMODYNAMICS

Damping of the Pulsatile Cardiac Output

The stroke volume issues at regular intervals from the ventricles and is associated with a bouncy pulse pressure. This pulsatile situation is smoothed out (damped) by a combination of arterial compliance and arteriolar resistance. Figure 3.16a depicts the situation to be found with very stiff (noncompliant) arteries, and Fig. 3.16b shows what effect the addition of more arterial compliance (less stiffness) has on arterial pressure waves. The mean pressure is unaffected in the new steady state by this increased compliance, hence our resistance calculation linking flow and mean pressure is still valid. The swings of arterial pressure, however, are smaller in the presence of a higher arterial compliance because the compliant artery effectively stores pressure energy during systole (ventricular contraction) and gives it back during diastole (ventricular relaxation). In this, the normal situation, the more constant pressure within arteries produces a more constant flow through the tissues.

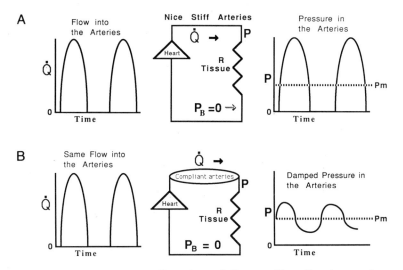

FIG. 3.16. **a:** Pressure profile mirrors inflow profile without compliance. **b:** Arterial compliance damps arterial pressure.

Effects of Varying Circulatory Parameters

We're now in a position to understand some of the effects of changing circulatory variables. Consider an increase in circulatory driving **pressure.** Unopposed by an increased resistance, the flow would simply increase (Eq. 3.12). Similarly, pushing a larger flow through an unchanged resistance will require a larger pressure gradient across the resistance. Increasing systemic arteriolar resistance in the face of continued tissue demands for blood flow will require higher driving pressures (hypertension).

A leakage path in parallel with normal tissue vascular resistance, termed an arteriovenous shunt, effectively lowers the **circulatory resistance** so much that mean arterial pressures will fall somewhat, and diastolic pressures may approach zero. Systolic pressures, on the other hand, may be somewhat higher than normal because of control mechanisms to be discussed later.

Increasing **heart rate** will increase cardiac output if stroke volume can be kept constant. This won't happen if **venous return** to the heart is not augmented concomitantly. The result will be tiny stroke volumes at more frequent intervals unless an arrangement is made with the venous system. More on this later.

An increase in **venous volume** will, if venous compliance is kept constant, produce an increase in venous pressure. This is one way to drive more blood into the heart and increase venous return. The extra water needed for this can be derived from the tissues as described below.

WORK OF CONTRACTION

How much work does the heart do while all this is going on? Figure 3.17a is a pressure–volume diagram of the left ventricle. The curve describes the path taken by pressure and volume during a single cardiac cycle. The details of this curve are discussed in Chapter 4. Here we wish to point out that the area enclosed by the curve represents the external work performed by the heart in a Carnot cycle, that is, it is equal to $\int PdV$. Those readers unfamiliar with such physiocochemical notions can easily verify that the units of this graphical area represent mechanical work: multiply pressure times volume and examine the result (e.g.: Newtons/m^2 $\times$ m^3 = Newtons $\times$ m = work). The bigger the area enclosed by the curve, the more external work the heart is doing per beat. We qualify work by calling it external (or perhaps useful) because, as will be discussed in Chapter 4, there are additional energy costs to be paid that don't serve to push the blood around the circulation.

It is important that you understand two basic ways in which this external work of the heart could be increased.

Figure 3.17b is an example of a situation in which the left ventricle is given the job of increasing its stroke volume while keeping arterial pressures normal. The net result is an increase in the pressure times volume product per beat. Because the contraction started from a higher than normal end diastolic volume, the muscle fibers were stretched more than usual at the start, and this situation is

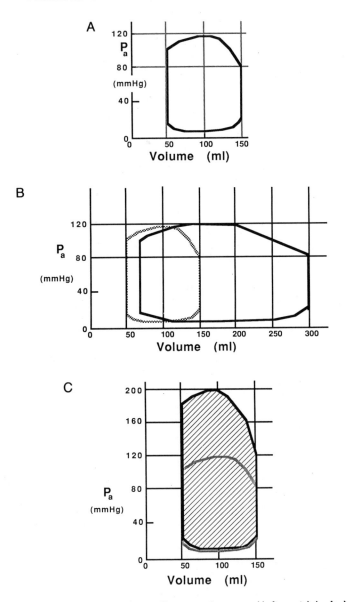

FIG. 3.17. **a:** Pressure–volume diagram of a normal left ventricle. **b:** Volume load. **c:** Pressure load.

often referred to as an increase in preload. The name preload actually derives from experiments performed on muscle strips (see Chapter 4) in which the strips are loaded (stressed, stretched) prior to stimulation. Preload can be calculated by the Laplace relationship (Eq. 3.16d). It is equivalent to the wall stress calculated for a point in the lower right hand corner of a ventricular pressure–volume diagram (Fig. 3.17a).

Fig. 3.17c shows another rather straightforward way to make the heart work harder: One can require the heart to generate higher pressures **after** it starts to contract. Again, the area of the pressure–volume plot is increased if a normal stroke volume is maintained. Clinicians often refer to this as an increased afterload on the heart because the unsuspecting heart muscle doesn't encounter the load until **after** it begins to contract. It is analogous to the additional load (stress) encountered by a muscle strip just after it begins contracting. Remember, however, that the real afterload on the heart is the additional stress that the ventricular wall has to develop to generate arterial pressures. As was discussed on pages 73–79, wall stress rises both with **pressure** and with the **size** of the heart and is inversely related to the thickness of the ventricle. Total load varies during ventricular systole and is the same as the wall stress calculated from the law of Laplace (Eq. 3.16d) for any systolic point on the ventricular pressure–volume curve. True afterload for a ventricle will be the total load minus the preload.

CAPILLARY FLUID EXCHANGE

Figure 3.18 is a simplified presentation of capillary fluid balance. Net hydrostatic capillary transmural pressure (P inside − P outside) tends to drive water outward all along the length of capillaries. The transmural pressure drops along the length of these vessels because of capillary resistance, so that it starts out at perhaps 35 mm Hg at the arteriolar end and declines to 7 mm Hg at the venular end. The tissue hydrostatic pressure component of this transmural pressure, tending to push the fluid back into the capillaries, will be on the order of 5 mm Hg. Lacking other forces, capillaries

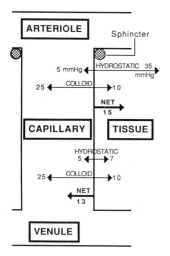

FIG. 3.18. Forces tending to cause filtration and reabsorption in a typical systemic capillary.

would leak fluid into the tissues throughout their entire length. This is prevented by plasma proteins which create a colloid osmotic pressure (also called oncotic pressure) of approximately 25 mm Hg, tending to draw fluid into the capillaries from the tissues. Proteins present in the extravascular fluid, on the other hand, will contribute roughly a 10-mm Hg pressure tending to suck fluid out of the capillaries. The net osmotic force is therefore $25 - 10 = 15$ mm Hg acting to keep fluid within capillaries. At the arteriolar end hydraulic forces are greater than osmotic and fluid will flow into the tissues bearing essential substances like glucose and oxygen. (Almost all exchange of gases, nutrients, electrolytes, and all other small molecules occurs by **diffusion** between capillaries and tissues, however.) By the time the venule is reached the situation is reversed and the declining hydrostratic pressure cannot prevent reentry of fluid into the circulation. Not all that leaves returns, however, and the slack is taken up by the lymphatics. The system depends upon lots of plasma protein (principally albumin) and an intact capillary endothelium.

Things that tend to produce excess tissue fluid (edema) are high venous pressures, blocked lymphatics, low plasma proteins, and protein leaks in the endothelium. Tending to retard the formation of edema are lower capillary pressures (often secondary to increased arteriolar resistance) and higher tissue hydrostatic pressures. For example, the progressively higher venous pressures associated with right-sided heart failure first produce ankle edema, then leg edema, and then even a backing up of tissue fluids into the peritoneal cavity (ascites).

QUESTIONS

Figure 3.19 is a graph of wall stress times wall thickness (S × h) versus radius (r) in a blood vessel. Use curves 1–4 and points A–E to answer **Questions 3.01–3.03.**

3.01. Of the points shown in the graph, which defines a state with the greatest ACTIVE tension times wall thickness?

a. A   d. D
b. B   e. E
c. C

3.02. The curve(s) representing the passive characteristics of the vessel is (are):

a. 1   d. 4
b. 2   e. 2, 3, and 4
c. 3

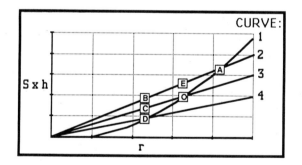

FIG. 3.19.   See Questions 3.01–3.03.

3.03. We shall use the same graph for a venule with different X and Y scales. Suppose that B is the normal operating point of a venule in the leg. If the sympathetic tone to that venule alone were to be completely shut off, its new operating point would most likely be:

a. A   d. D
b. B   e. E
c. C

In a patient suspected of having pulmonary hypertension and a septal defect, oxygen consumption is 250 ml/min, STPD, and oxygen capacity of hemoglobin is 200 ml O_2/L blood. Ignore the dissolved oxygen for the purposes of these questions. Assume that this person's lungs are oxygenating blood normally as it passes through them. Use Fig. 3.20 and the pressures and oxygen contents in various locations as specified below to answer **Questions 3.04 and 3.05.**

	Mean pressure (mm Hg)	O_2 content (ml O_2/L blood)
Pulmonary artery	105	150
Left atrium	5	Not measured
Brachial artery	100	183.3
Right atrium	10	150

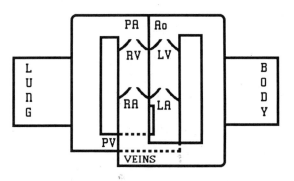

FIG. 3.20.   See Questions 3.04 and 3.05.

3.04. Flow through the defect (shunt flow) in L/min is closest to:

a. 2   d. 5
b. 2.5   e. 7.5
c. 3

3.05. If, during exercise, the peripheral vascular resistance decreased more than the left ventricular output increased while the pulmonary vascular resistance remained the same, one would expect (choose from a–e below):

	a.	b.	c.	d.	e.
Shunt flow	↑	↑	↑	↓	↓
Aortic % sat.	↑	Same	↓	↓	↓

A 24-year-old male with increasing shortness of breath was admitted to UCSF for cardiac catheterization. Use the following data to answer **Questions 3.06–3.09.**

$\dot{V}_{O_2}$	160 ml/min, STPD
[Hemoglobin]	181 g/L
O_2 capacity	246 ml O_2/L
Hematocrit	57%
Heart rate	92 beats/min

Location	O_2 Content (ml O_2/L)	Blood pressure (mm Hg) Sys./dias.	Mean
Inf. vena cava	165	—/—	2
Sup. vena cava	165	—/—	2
Right atrium	165	—/—	2
Right ventricle	180	112/2	—
Pulmonary artery	180	110/80	90
Left atrium	228	—/—	3
Left ventricle	210	122/2	—
Brachial artery	210	120/70	85

3.06. The systemic blood flow in L/min is closest to:

a. 2.55   d. 5.35
b. 3.33   e. 8.90
c. 3.55

3.07. The pulmonary blood flow in L/min is closest to:

a. 2.55   d. 5.35
b. 3.33   e. 8.90
c. 3.55

3.08. Arterial O_2 content is 210 ml/L instead of normal most likely because of:

a. Low O_2 consumption.
b. Abnormally bad distribution of $\dot{V}_A/\dot{Q}$ in the lungs.
c. Myocardial failure resulting in inadequate cardiac output.
d. Elevated [Hb] combined with an intracardiac left-to-right shunt.
e. Elevated [Hb] combined with an intracardiac right-to-left shunt.

3.09. This patient's data indicate an:

a. Intraatrial right-to-left shunt only.
b. Intraventricular right-to-left shunt only.
c. Intraventricular left-to-right shunt only.
d. Intraventricular bidirectional shunt with more $\dot{Q}$ going R → L than L → R.
e. Intraventricular bidirectional shunt with more $\dot{Q}$ going L → R than R → L.

In essence, the circulation of kidneys can be considered to consist of two vascular resistances in series. There is a preglomerular resistance (primarily the afferent arterioles) and a postglomerular resistance (primarily the efferent arterioles and the peritubular capillaries), with the glomerular capillaries in between these two resistances. For the purposes of these questions, please ignore glomerular filtration, tubular reabsorption, and resistance along the glomerular capillaries themselves. Use the data below to answer **Questions 3.10–3.13.**

	Period A	Period B
Mean renal arterial pressure	100 mm Hg	100 mm Hg
Preglomerular resistance	R1	2 (R1)
Mean glomerular capillary pressure	70 mm Hg	???
Postglomerular resistance	R2	R2
Renal venous pressure	10 mm Hg	10 mm Hg
Renal blood flow	1.5 L/min	???

3.10. In period A, the preglomerular resistance is what fraction of the total?

  a. 1/4   d. 2/3
  b. 1/3   e. 3/4
  c. 1/2

3.11. What is the total renal vascular resistance in period A?

  a. 67 mm Hg/(L/min)   d. 0.167 (L/min)/mm Hg
  b. 60 mm Hg/(L/min)   e. 0.150 (L/min)/mm Hg
  c. 30 mm Hg/(L/min)

3.12. In period B preglomerular resistance is twice what is was in period A, while postglomerular resistance and arterial and venous pressures are the same. Mean glomerular capillary pressure in mm Hg in period B is closest to:

  a. 85   d. 55
  b. 70   e. 40
  c. 60

3.13. In period B, the renal blood flow in L/min is closest to:

  a. 2.000   d. 1.125
  b. 1.500   e. 0.750
  c. 1.250

The hepatic circulation is somewhat complex because there are two arterial supplies (the mesenteric and hepatic arteries) and two capillary beds in series (the intestines and the liver). Flow from the hepatic artery merges with that from the portal vein in the anastomosing capillary bed of the liver. Use the summary of the anatomy, average vascular pressures (in mm Hg), and flows in ml/min in a normal resting adult (Fig. 3.21) for **Questions 3.14 and 3.15.**

3.14. The vascular resistance of the total splanchnic circulation (mesenteric and hepatic routes taken together, ending at the right atrium), in mm Hg/(L/min) is:

a. 65   d. 90
b. 69   e. 390
c. 88

3.15. Which of the following vascular segments has the highest resistance?

a. Aorta via hepatic artery to liver capillaries.
b. Aorta via mesenteric artery to intestinal capillaries.
c. Intestinal capillaries to portal vein.
d. Portal vein to liver capillaries.
e. Liver capillaries to right atrium.

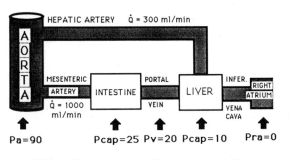

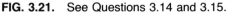

FIG. 3.21.   See Questions 3.14 and 3.15.

ANSWERS

3.01. d. Curve 1 depicts the passive characteristics of the vessel in question, while curves 2, 3, and 4 are graphs of Laplace's law for each of three different pressures. Points A, O, and B represent equilibrium points which could be achieved if the vessel were to behave completely passively when subjected to the three different pressures. Points C, D, and E represent possible equilibria under conditions in which the smooth muscle in the wall of the vessel is providing some active tension as well. In fact, the point's vertical distance above the passive tension curve is equal to the active component.

3.02. a. See explanation immediately above.

3.03. a. The operating point **B** represents a situation in which there is considerable sympathetic tone providing considerable active tension. If that sympathetic tone were to be removed, the vessel must expand. What path will it take? The venular pressure, which generated Laplace's law curve 2, will have no reason to change as a result of this one venule in the leg losing its sympathetic tone. Thus, the new equilibrium point must occur at the intersection of the passive curve and curve 2.

3.04. b. The O_2 content in the left atrium, while not given in the table, is actually known to be approximately 200 ml O_2/L blood since you are told that the lungs are oxygenating the blood normally and that the O_2 capacity of the hemoglobin is 200 ml O_2/L blood. Thus, one can calculate the systemic flow to be 250 ml O_2/min/ 33.3 ml O_2/L blood = 7.5 L/min, and the pulmonary flow to be 250/50 = 5 L/min. The shunt flow must therefore be = 2.5 L/min.

3.05. c. The drop in O_2 content between the left atrium and the brachial artery reveals a right-to-left shunt, through an interatrial or interventricular defect. What drives $\dot{Q}$ through a defect is a difference in pressure on the two sides of the defect. In this case, the pressure in the right atrium is higher than that in the left, and the pressure in the pulmonary artery is higher than that in the brachial artery (and thus, the pressure in the right ventricle is most likely higher than that in the left). As always, the driving pressure ($P_{driving}$) depends on the product of $\dot{Q}$ and resistance (R). If the systemic R decreases greatly while the systemic $\dot{Q}$ only increases somewhat, the systemic $P_{driving}$ must decrease. Practically speaking, this means that P_{Ao} must decrease and thus that P_{LV} must also decrease. These decreases amount to a decrease of afterload on the left ventricle, so the filling pressures in the left atrium must also decrease. Thus the pressure gradient across the defect, already favoring right-to-left $\dot{Q}$ in the control state, must now be increased. If the right-to-left $\dot{Q}$ increases, then the aortic O_2 saturation must decrease.

3.06. c. The Fick principle again, but use care about which values one uses. Systemic flow $= \dot{V}_{O2}/(Ca_{O2} - C\bar{v}_{O2}) = (160$ ml $O_2/min)/(210 - 165$ ml O_2/L blood$) = 3.55$ L blood/min.

3.07. b. See answer to Question 3.06.

3.08. e. Normal arterial blood is essentially fully saturated with O_2, yielding an O_2 content of about 200 ml O_2/L blood. This patient, because of his high hematocrit, has a high O_2 capacity of his hemoglobin (246 ml O_2/L blood). If there were no right-to-left shunt, his arterial blood would be expected to have an O_2 content near 246. The shunt lowers it to only 210 ml O_2/L blood.

3.09. d. The O_2 content of right atrial blood increases as it passes into the right ventricle, and the O_2 content of left atrial blood decreases as it passes into the left ventricle. These two changes in content can only happen if the shunt flow is bidirectional. As the systemic flow $>>$ pulmonary flow, the right–left component must be greater than the left–right component.

3.10. c. An exercise in the use of Ohm's law in a system of resistances in series. $P_{driving} = R \times \dot{Q}$. In a series system such as this, the $\dot{Q}$ through all parts is necessarily equal. Thus, the $P_{driving}$ in any given segment depends, for a given $\dot{Q}$, only upon the R of that segment. As the $P_{driving}$ across the preglomerular resistance is 30 mm Hg and that across the total resistance is 90 mm Hg, the preglomerular resistance must be ⅓ the total resistance.

3.11. b. Ohm's law again. $R = P_{driving}/\dot{Q} = (90 - 10)$ mm Hg/(1.5 L/min) = 60 mm Hg/(L/min).

3.12. d. See answer to Question 3.10. In period A, the preglomerular resistance was ½ of the postglomerular resistance. In period B, they must be equal. Thus, ½ of the $P_{driving}$ of 90 (or 45 mm Hg) must occur across each resistance. $100 - 45 = 55$.

3.13. d. As the total resistance has increased to 4/3 what it was in period A, the $\dot{Q}$ must be 3/4 what it was.

3.14. b. The overall $\dot{Q}$ is the sum of the two flows or 1.3 L/min. $R = P_{driving}/\dot{Q} = 90/1.3 = 69$ mm Hg/(L/min).

3.15. a. One must plug in the $P_{driving}/\dot{Q}$ for each of the vascular segments.

4

The Heart as a Pump

INTRODUCTION

This section describes the events of the cardiac cycle and shows how the heart functions independent of external control mechanisms. It distinguishes between the Frank–Starling effect and contractility and shows how our bodies use these two inherently different ways of increasing the energy of contraction.

BACK TO BASICS: ISOLATED MUSCLE STRIPS

Purpose

Before we study the intact heart we will examine the properties of intact linear strips of heart muscle, such as thin isolated heart papillary muscles, in order to show that one can increase the force of cardiac muscle contraction in two different ways:

1. by increasing the **initial length** of the muscle strip prior to producing a contraction (This is related to the **Frank–Starling** mechanism.); and
2. by using other (usually chemical) means (This associated increase of force is called an increase in **contractility.**).

Both of these mechanisms may be deranged in disease, and both respond to treatment.

99

Observations

Connect a cat right ventricular papillary muscle (1 × 10 mm) to a force-measuring transducer in a superfusing bath in which it can be electrically stimulated. Stretch the resting muscle to different lengths and measure the maximum force developed by the passive stretching alone. The results should look like the lowest curve in Fig. 4.1 which is called the passive length–tension curve. A similar result follows from stretching certain kinds of inert springs. Note the similarity to Fig. 3.13b, in which the passive stretching of another kind of muscle (in the vessel wall) is expressed by stress (a force per cross-sectional area) on the Y axis versus a linear stretching dimension (radius) on the X axis.

Now repeat the stretching process, but this time electrically stimulate the muscle so that it develops an additional active force at each fixed, stretched length, and again measure this force. Such an active length–tension relationship is plotted as the upper curve in Fig. 4.1.

This exercise demonstrates that higher force development results from such muscles if contractions start from longer initial lengths. Note that you can also overstretch the muscle to the point where developed tension decreases with further stretching.

Now repeat the experiments in the presence of some norepinephrine, which will interact with beta$_1$ receptors in heart muscle and produce an increase in contractility. The results are plotted in Fig. 4.2 as the uppermost dashed curve. The conclusion is that **at any fixed initial length** one can get an increase in force development

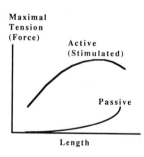

FIG. 4.1. Isometric contractions of a muscle strip.

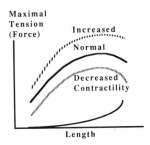
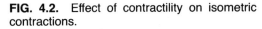

FIG. 4.2. Effect of contractility on isometric contractions.

by exposing the muscle to norepinephrine. Increased force can therefore be obtained by both length-dependent and contractility-dependent mechanisms.

If we bathe the muscle with a pentobarbital-containing solution, we will decrease its contractility (lower dashed curve), and thus decrease its ability to generate force at any given initial length.

The above experiments were done in an isometric fashion, that is, with muscle length kept constant during contraction. What happens during isoload experiments in which a fixed load (weight) is lifted by the muscle while length is allowed to change?

The experimental findings are usually plotted on a force–velocity diagram like Fig. 4.3. Here the maximum velocity of the contracting muscle is plotted against the concomitant force developed for one particular preload and varying additional loads (afterloads) during contraction. This curve meets the force (X) axis at a velocity equal to zero, because afterload plus preload is so great that the muscle can't move it. At the same stretching preload, but with progressively lighter afterloads, the muscle is able to contract with increasing

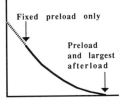

FIG. 4.3. Vary afterload.

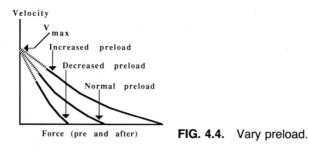

FIG. 4.4. Vary preload.

velocity. The fastest measureable velocity is recorded when there is no afterload, that is, when preload is the total load.

A larger preload gives the uppermost line in Fig. 4.4, producing a larger X intercept. A lower preload will do the reverse. Nonlinear extrapolations of these curves toward the velocity axis often tend to intersect near a common point V_{max}, or maximum velocity.

If we now bathe the muscle of these latter force–velocity experiments in norepinephrine to increase contractility, we can move the constant preload curve of Fig. 4.3 upward, and produce a higher V_{max} as in Fig. 4.5. Lowering contractility with pentobarbital produces a lower V_{max}, and so V_{max} appears to be a good indicator of contractility.

Conclusions

We hope you will conclude from these findings that a contracting muscle can develop more force in two seemingly different ways: (1) by being stretched to longer initial lengths, and (2) by other

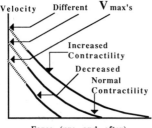

FIG. 4.5. Vary contractility.

(usually chemical) means. We will associate the term contractility **only** with these latter, non-length-dependent mechanisms. While some authors do not adhere to this restricted use of contractility, the underlying physiology remains the same.

Reservations

Muscles act as if their pure contractile elements (CE) are arranged so as to stretch series elastic (SE) ''springs'' and parallel elastic (PE) ''springs'' within the muscle (Fig. 4.6). When one takes this into account and plots the velocity, not of the muscle itself but of the CE, V_{max}s become a bit more coherent. Note, however, that such an analysis depends on the particular model of how the CE is hooked up to the SE and PE. Most recent experiments, heavily involving computer control and more carefully assessing experimental artifacts, have shown that there is no unique V_{max} corresponding to a given state of contractility. Thus, the cardiac physiological

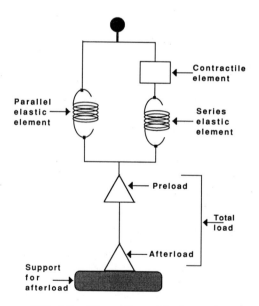

FIG. 4.6. Maxwell model of muscle.

literature reflects a period during which V_{max} was the preferred indicator of contractility. Currently, a parameter derived from ventricular pressure–volume plots is favored over V_{max}. More of this later.

EVENTS OF THE CARDIAC CYCLE AND THEIR TIME RELATIONSHIPS

Figure 4.7, based on a well-known diagram from Wiggers (1), will be seen in some form in every textbook dealing with the heart. It offers an excellent visual means of displaying heart happenings as seen from various viewpoints. Refer to this figure as you read the following discussion.

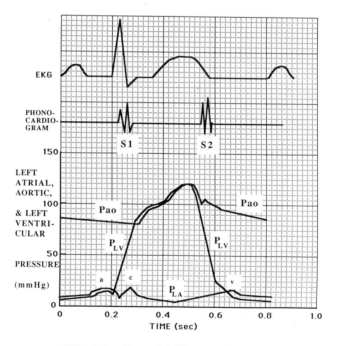

FIG. 4.7.   (Pseudo) Wiggers diagram.

The EKG

The repetitive excitation process initiates each cycle of contractile events. The electrocardiogram (EKG) gives a reliable picture of this excitation process, and we should relate the mechanical events we see elsewhere to this time scale.

The P wave reports the spread of the depolarization wave (excitation) through the atrial muscle. The origin of this wave is in the sinoatrial (SA) node, but such a small localized process cannot be seen from the usual EKG leads. Similarly, after the atria have been excited, the passage of the depolarization wave through the tiny atrioventricular (AV) node into the ventricles is invisible to us, unless we use leads that actually touch this structure. It is certain that atrial excitation must precede atrial contraction if the latter is to occur at all. Therefore, P waves must occur before atrial squeezes.

On the usual EKG tracing, we don't see much of note following the P wave until the muscle of the ventricle starts depolarizing, generating the so-called QRS complex. By the time this starts, the AV node, the common bundle of His, and much of the Purkinje system have all been depolarized.

Electrical peace ensues as the entire ventricle has been "shocked" from a polarized to an essentially depolarized state, and the ST segment of the EKG is being inscribed. Mechanically, ventricular muscle contraction has begun **following** the excitation process. It continues on in an active fashion until some milliseconds past the inscription of the peak of the T wave of the EKG, which reports the ventricular repolarization process.

During the ST segment, calcium conductance, $g_{Ca^{2+}}$, is high and the influx of Ca^{2+} triggers contraction. As the T wave is written $g_{Ca^{2+}}$ becomes low and muscle Ca^{2+} pumps effectively remove this ion from the contractile apparatus, allowing the muscle to relax.

So, the excitation process has produced simultaneous contractions of both atria followed by simultaneous contractions of both ventricles. These events can be seen in the pressure, volume, and sound recordings described below.

Left Ventricular Pressure, Volume, and Heart Sounds

Introduce the tip of a catheter into a brachial artery and then retrograde via the aorta and aortic valve (wait for systole) into the left ventricle. Hook a pressure transducer to its end, and you can follow the pressure history of ventricular contraction. A similar story, on a somewhat attenuated pressure scale, is being told on the right side of the heart in the other ventricle.

Very likely as the left atrium contracts and sends the **last** portion of cardiac input into the relaxed and almost filled left ventricle a little pressure wave will be seen within the ventricle. This atrial "kick" thus marks end diastole and fills the ventricle to its end diastolic volume (EDV), the largest volume it will attain during the whole cycle. Occasionally this process is associated with an audible fourth heart sound. This sound is rarely heard in healthy individuals.

The ventricle in its turn then contracts, raising ventricular pressure above that of the left atrium, thereby slamming its back door, the mitral valve, and shaking the entire thoracic house with the first heart sound. There are sometimes two components to this sound, with the first being contributed by closure of the mitral valve. The first heart sound is the loudest and is transmitted best where the heart touches the chest wall: at the apex of the heart and near the sternum.

LV pressure rises rapidly in the ensuing phase of isovolumetric contraction. In general, the healthier or more vigorous the heart is, the more rapid will be this rate of rise, i.e., dP/dt is higher. The phase is called isovolumetric because both the mitral and aortic valves are shut and a constant volume is trapped within the heart.

Eventually pressure in the ventricle becomes greater than in the aorta, and this pressure gradient opens the aortic valve, pushing blood out of the heart into the arterial system. This beginning of the systolic ejection phase (end of isovolumetric contraction phase) is normally a quiet process. Opening a heart valve makes little noise unless it sticks a bit, there is a larger than normal rush of blood through it, or a small stenotic opening resists blood flow through it.

Pressure rises still more as the ventricle empties part of its contents. Maximal pressure in the ventricle is normally the same as is achieved in the arterial system, 120 mm Hg, because there is normally very little resistance to flow between heart and aorta.

During this ejection phase, the heart's motion in the thorax appears strange: The base of the heart, where the great veins and arteries are connected, actually moves downward and to the left toward the relatively immobile apex. It is claimed that this downward pulling of the open aortic and pulmonic valves around the initially immobile columns of blood in the outflow tracts is an aid in getting blood out of the heart.

As the Ca^{2+} supply to the actin–myosin contractile mechanism is depleted by the action of Ca^{2+} pumps during repolarization the muscle begins to relax. This doesn't happen suddenly in square-wave fashion, but is a smooth backing-off of active muscle tension.

At a certain point ventricular pressure falls below aortic pressure and blood would flow back into the ventricle except that the first rearward rush abruptly closes the aortic valve. Again, a valve closing produces a noise, the second heart sound. Although the ventricle is still developing force, this moment is often called the end systolic point. We will return to this when discussing contractility, pages 113, 115, 119–120.

The ventricle now contains its smallest volume ever: end systolic volume (ESV). Both ventricular valves are shut, trapping blood inside the chamber while the heart continues its relaxation. Beyond this point, as the contractile fibers generate decreasing force, ventricular pressure falls during the so-called isometric relaxation phase. The heart is still contracting, but doing so less forcefully.

Eventually ventricular pressure falls below that in the large blood pool sitting in the now distended left atrium and pulmonary veins. The pressure gradient across the mitral valve pushes the valve open and pours a substantial fraction of the subsequent stroke volume into the ventricle in what is called the rapid filling phase of diastole.

It should be emphasized that pressure is still falling during all of this phase because the ventricle is still relaxing: that is, force development is still present but is heading toward zero.

At the very end of relaxation, the partially distended ventricle has reached the end of its "crumpled paper bag" configuration and suddenly begins to resist further easy filling from continued venous return into the venoatrial-ventricular pool. If the heart is reasonably large and has a normal stroke volume and compliance, the end of the rapid filling phase will be heard through the stethoscope as a thud (the third heart sound). Many normal young people, athletes with large stroke volumes, and people with large hearts in failure will have this sound, but not all people will.

After this event, venous return from the lungs continues to fill the ventricle, but at a slower rate. This is appropriately termed the slow ventricular filling phase or diastasis. It is characterized by a progressive increase of ventricular pressure to perhaps 5 to 8 mm Hg. Near the very end of diastole the atria contract, starting the whole cycle over again.

Aortic Pressure

Let's look at pressure in the **aorta** during this cycle because the aorta is directly hooked up to the ventricle. The aorta is separated from ventricular happenings in late diastole by the closed aortic valve. During this diastolic phase, blood is leaving the aorta to supply the various organs, and pressure is inevitably and relentlessly falling toward (but not reaching) 7 mm Hg. This restful state is interrupted as the aortic valve bursts open and blood is ejected out of the heart. While the aortic valve is open aortic pressure tends to follow ventricular pressure quite closely, lagging behind it very slightly in time because of the inertia of the flowing blood. In other words, the aortic pressure tracing is shifted ever so slightly behind the ventricular record in time, due to part of the aortic blood energy being momentarily tied up in kinetic (flow) as opposed to potential (pressure) energy.

The compliant (stretchable) arterial system accepts the ventricle's stroke volume and even attempts to return some of it to the pump as ventricular pressure starts to drop late in the systolic ejection phase. This attempted backward flow is thwarted by the aortic valve closing, however, and the blood, in bouncing off the valve, probably creates the dicrotic notch of the arterial pressure wave, which marks the end systolic point.

Hereafter the pressure declines exponentially toward 7 mm Hg, waiting to be interrupted by the reopening of the aortic valve. This interruption usually occurs at a pressure of around 80 mm Hg, giving a blood pressure of 120 over 80. Should the next aortic opening be delayed by a missed heart beat or even a very slow heart rate, this diastolic pressure will be allowed to fall to a lower value. Diastolic pressures will also be lower when blood runs out of the large arteries faster than normal or when the arterial system is less compliant than normal.

Atrial and Large Vein Pressures

When the atria squeeze immediately after the P wave they raise pressure locally and farther back in the connected large veins. In all these structures this pressure wave is called the a (for atrial) wave.

The next bump on the atrial pressure curve is caused by ventricular contraction. This occurs because the valve between the atria and ventricles is thin and flexible and transmits a good c (for contraction) wave back into the atriovenous system.

The last bump is called the v wave. Once the atrioventricular valves have been shut by ventricular contraction, there is no place for continuing venous return to go. It stretches the venoatrial reservoir, raising its pressure, and generating the **upstroke** of the v wave. The atrioventricular valves then open because ventricular pressure has dropped to below that in the atria, and the blood has a still-relaxing, low-pressure cavity to flow into. Atrial pressure accordingly begins to drop, inscribing the downslope of the v wave.

The peak of the v thus represents the moment at which the atrioventricular valves open, and also the point where the phase of rapid ventricular filling begins.

The a, c, and v waves (note the fortunate alphabetic order) are found in both atria and both (systemic and pulmonary) venous systems. All three waves can be recognized in the neck veins of most subjects.

EVENTS OF THE CARDIAC CYCLE AS SEEN ON THE
PRESSURE–VOLUME DIAGRAM

Let's look at these same events on a pressure–volume plot of the left ventricle (Fig. 4.8a). Start at the lower left-hand corner of the loop. The mitral valve has just opened because left ventricular pressure has finally fallen below that in the left atrium. In the

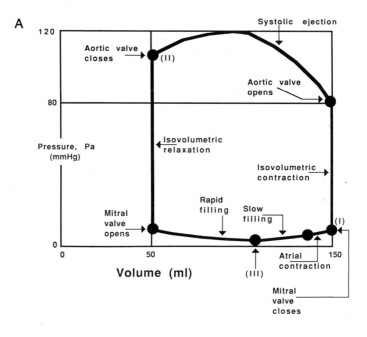

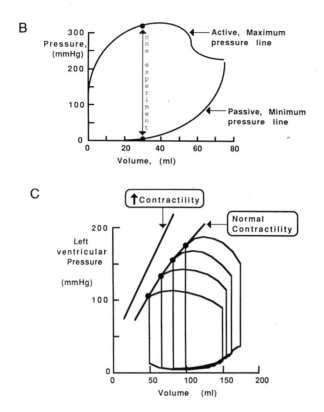

FIG. 4.8. **a:** Left ventricular pressure–volume diagram. **b:** Isovolumetric contractions of a dog heart at different volumes. (From E. H. Starling's Linacre Lecture.) **c:** Contractility as defined by plots of end systolic points.

ensuing rapid filling phase blood rushes into the left ventricle as it continues to relax, allowing an increase in volume and yet a concomitant decrease in pressure.

At the end of this phase, the ventricle reaches a kind of elastic limit and a low-pitched sound (third heart sound, III) is often heard, similar to that heard on blowing up a paper bag.

The slow filling phase is driven by continuing venous return and contributes only one-fourth to one-third of the cardiac input. Note that pressure rises during this volume increase.

This relatively long phase is terminated by the contraction of the atrium, which sends a small and final amount of blood into the ventricle as it slightly increases ventricular pressure.

Ventricular contraction follows, closing the mitral valve, and thereby producing the first heart sound (I). Pressure then rises while ventricular volume remains constant at end diastolic volume, during the period known as isovolumetric contraction.

When ventricular pressure rises high enough, it pushes the aortic valve open. Aortic pressure starts to rise from this, its lowest point, also known as the aortic diastolic pressure.

During the following phase of systolic ejection ventricular and aortic pressures both rise and fall together because these two chambers are connected by the open aortic valve. Ventricular volume has been decreasing ever since the aortic valve opened and continues to do so until this same valve closes again, creating the second heart sound (II). Note that when this valve closes, ventricular pressure is higher than when it opens on the next cycle. This has to be because aortic pressure falls during this interval. Aortically speaking, the closure of the aortic valve marks the end of systole. Some authors, particularly those favoring a particular index of contractility based on the ventricular pressure–volume diagram, term this the end systolic point. Its importance will be discussed later.

During the next phase, known as isovolumetric relaxation, the ventricle is really still contracting because, although pressure is falling, muscle fibers in the ventricle are still developing some tension. This contraction will continue until some time in the rapid filling phase.

When ventricular pressure has fallen low enough, however, the mitral valve is forced open by the pressure that has been building in the left atrium, and we are back to where we started.

HOW THE ISOLATED, INTACT HEART WORKS WITHOUT CONTROLS

Studying the mechanics of ventricular muscle strips is an abstract process in which one can see only dimly what actually happens in the intact animal. Physiologists have long worked with animal experimental models of intermediate complexity, hoping to retain some of the simplicity of muscle strip work while avoiding the complications of neural and hormonal control mechanisms belonging to the animal. The Starling heart–lung preparation discussed in this section represents one such level of abstraction. Much of what happens in this preparation happens in the intact animal as well.

Measures of Preload, Afterload, and Contractility in the Intact Heart

Preload in the intact heart is defined as the passive force per cross-sectional area (stress) present in muscle fiber bundles before they contract. Without measuring this force directly researchers have often used other variables that reflect the force–length relationships of the myocardium just before contraction to calculate it. Thus, end diastolic ventricular diameter (from ultrasonic measurements), end diastolic volume (from ultrasonic and angiographic measurements), and end diastolic ventricular pressure (from catheters pushed into the ventricles) have been used commonly to calculate the preloading of the ventricle just before contraction. One gets estimates of chamber radius, wall thickness, and transmural pressure, and then uses the Laplace relationship (Eq. 3.16d) to calculate the preload (equals wall stress). The tendency in clinical situations is to regard a variable such as right atrial pressure, P_{RA}, as the preload on the right ventricular myocardium, but this neglects the important contribution of ventricular size to its preload.

Afterload (related to active tension development) is more difficult to define and measure in the intact heart. Implanted strain gauges can record ventricular wall stress as the muscle contracts, but their placement involves difficult and invasive surgery. As in the case of preload, pressure and dimensional measurements can be used in Laplace's law to calculate the wall stress during a contraction. Subtracting the relevant preload from this total wall stress would give us the afterload, but there is no satisfactory way to choose a preload to match a given afterload. For example, the preload of an athlete's heart will be large, reflecting the very large end diastolic volume, and yet the total load or stress at the closing of the aortic valve during systole may be even lower than the preload if aortic pressure is low.

Clinically, the **total** load at any point during systole is usually termed **afterload,** purposely neglecting the fact that some kind of preload should ideally be subtracted. Previously, clinicians equated afterload with pressure alone, disregarding the contribution to wall stress that comes from ventricular radius. Acknowledging the law of Laplace, modern clinical treatment of heart failure attempts to keep the ventricle from becoming too large, and thus tries to lower this particular contribution to wall stress.

Contractility in the intact heart measures the ability of the heart muscle to do stroke work independent of changes in initial fiber length. We wish to emphasize this independence because, as you will see from the discussion of the Frank–Starling effect below, the heart is capable of increasing its work output simply because its fibers are stretched. It is obvious that the heart could increase its total work per time (i.e., minute work) by merely increasing the number of beats per minute. Such an increase in work output is also excluded from increases in contractility, which deal with stroke work alone. Experiments designed to assess increases in contractility therefore must keep heart rate and the precontraction myocardial stretch constant while measuring stroke work. This is hard to do in isolated papillary muscle experiments; it is even more difficult to accomplish in the intact animal or patient in whom end diastolic volume often changes as experimental variables are manipulated.

Putting these objections aside for now, consider that an increase in contractility means an increase in work per stroke at a constant initial fiber length. It could manifest itself as the ability to put out a larger stroke volume at an unchanged mean aortic pressure or to put out the same stroke volume against an increased mean aortic pressure. Keep in mind that end diastolic volume (initial fiber stretch = preload) must remain constant during these changes.

Contractility and the Pressure–Volume Diagram

Figure 4.8b comes from Ernest Starling's work just after the turn of the century. Otto Frank had produced similar curves somewhat earlier. On this special pressure–volume diagram of a dog's left ventricle are plotted two curves: a lower passive one and an upper active one. It is not the same kind of single pressure–volume loop shown in Fig. 4.8a. Rather, it presents the results of a large number of experiments in which the heart had to work against different afterloads (produced by varying vascular resistance). On the upper (active) curve are plotted the maximal values of systolic pressure from different individual contractions versus the end diastolic volume associated with each pressure. On the lower (passive) curve are plotted the end diastolic pressures associated with these same end diastolic volumes.

Figure 4.8c is the modern version of this old plot. In order to characterize contractility, interest has been shifted to the upper, active curve which now plots **end systolic pressure** rather than maximal systolic pressure versus the actual volume at which the pressure is achieved. For many mammalian hearts this plot of end-systolic points turns out to be nearly a straight line. It is handy because its slope is a reasonable index of myocardial contractility. Authors using this concept are a bit fuzzy about their definition of the end-systolic point, but it is probably fair to take it as the point when the aortic valve closes. It is thus an aortic definition of the end of systole because the ventricle still has some important relaxing to do before active tension has actually fallen to zero.

On Fig. 4.8 we have plotted several cardiac cycles in the traditional manner to give you some feeling for how the slope of the isocontractility line of end-systolic points remains reasonably constant during volume loading or volume deprivation. In this situation, contractility is supposed to stay constant as well. Changes in arteriolar resistance are also said not to move the line, in keeping with the idea that contractility should be independent of this circulatory parameter.

External Work, Wall Stress, and the Tension–Time Index

As we discussed earlier (pages 86–88), the external stroke work done by the heart, as manifested in the integral of PdV or approximated by mean ejection pressure × stroke volume, is not the whole story. Insofar as contractility and useful propulsion of blood are concerned, stroke work adequately describes what the heart can do for the circulation. However, it has a hidden load to bear in that maintaining high wall stresses (tensions) requires additional energy consumption. Thus, a heart will consume more substrate (break down more adenosine triphosphate) when it has to work at higher pressures, independent of the pressure × stroke volume product. Because energy supplies are limited there will usually be a trade-off, and the heart will be forced to waste pure stress-producing energy at the expense of useful external work. You may remember from the Laplace relationship that for a given transmural pressure, wall stress is proportional to the radius of the structure. Because blood pressures are reasonably constant in many physiological and pathological contexts, being big-hearted means doing more useless work.

A term used in describing part of this useless energy expenditure is the time–tension index, and it is often calculated by multiplying average ventricular **pressure** during systolic ejection by the systolic time. As you must realize from the foregoing discussion, this index neglects the considerable effect of changing ventricular size on wall stress (tension). The real message from this section is: Working at high volumes and high pressures imposes an extra load on the heart and detracts from its ability to do useful external work.

The Uncontrolled Heart: The Starling Heart–Lung Preparation

A traditional and yet up-to-date experimental model of how the uncontrolled circulation works is given by the Starling heart–lung preparation (Fig. 4.9). Indeed, physiologists and clinicians are today still applying some of the ideas inherent in this work performed

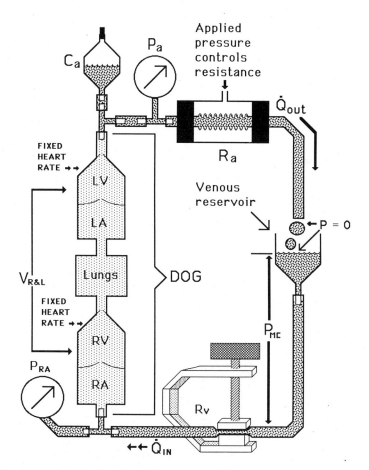

FIG. 4.9. The Starling heart–lung preparation.
Independent variables:
  Ra, arteriolar plus capillary resistance;
  P_{MC}, venous reservoir pressure, mean circulatory pressure;
  Rv, venous resistance (considered fixed here).
Intermediate dependent variables:
  $\dot{Q}_{in}$, cardiac input, venous return (usually not measured);
  $\dot{Q}_{out}$, cardiac output;
  $V_{R\&L}$, combined ventricular volumes;
  $\bar{P}a$, mean arterial pressure;
  $\bar{P}_{RA}$, mean right atrial pressure.
Final dependent variables:
  EDV, end diastolic volume, largest $V_{R\&L}$;
  V_S, stroke volume = $\dot{Q}_{out}$/rate;
  W_S, stroke work = Pa × V_S.
Important features:
  Chest is open (intrapleural pressure = atmospheric).
  Pericardium is removed and no longer limits ventricular volume.
  Extrinsic nervous and hormonal circulatory controls are removed.
  Heart rate is fixed.
  Contractility is constant.

just after the turn of the century. In this preparation only the heart
and lungs of a dog are allowed to survive. The rest of the dog,
deprived of circulating blood, dies, including all of the systemic
control mechanisms from baroreceptors and chemoreceptors to the
neural and hormonal means of controlling heart rate, heart contractility, arteriolar tone, and venous tone. By adding back selected components to the now abbreviated circulation, Starling was able to show
what the heart could do on its own, freed of complicating reflex
mechanisms. We shall begin by discussing the determinants of
venous return (cardiac **input**), a little emphasized topic in older
textbooks. Next we'll look at cardiac **output** as we describe the
Frank–Starling effect per se. Then we will bring input and output
together.

Venous Return (Cardiac Input) versus Atrial Pressure: The Input Curve

What Forces Drive Venous Return?

In the Starling heart–lung preparation, what causes blood to flow
into the right atrium? Figures 4.9 and 4.10 and the notion of hydraulic
resistance (pages 70–73) tell us. The driving force for this flow is
the pressure difference between the upraised venous reservoir [con-
tributing mean circulatory pressure (P_{MC})] and the pressure in the
right atrium (P_{RA}). These chambers differ in pressure because of
the venous resistance (Rv) lying between them. In the heart–lung
preparation, a screw clamp serves this function. The variables can
be related in Ohm's law as in Fig. 4.10 or plotted in the fashion
of Guyton as in Fig. 4.11.

$$\overline{P}_{RA} \bullet \sim\!\!\sim\!\!\sim\!\!\sim\!\!\sim \bullet P_{mc} \qquad \leftarrow\leftarrow\leftarrow \dot{Q}_{IN}$$

$$\dot{Q}_{IN} = \frac{Pmc - \overline{P}_{RA}}{Rv}$$

FIG. 4.10. Determinants of venous return.

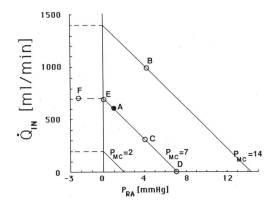

FIG. 4.11. Venous return (cardiac input) curve.

Effect of Raising Mean Circulatory Pressure P_{MC}

Clearly, raising the level of the reservoir will raise the P_{MC} on the right-hand side of the Rv and force more blood through the resistance into the right atrium. The heart will usually accept this and eventually match its output to its new input, experiencing a higher P_{RA} in the process. Such a maneuver is represented graphically in Fig. 4.11 by a shift from the normal operating point A to point B on a new venous return curve characterized by a new and higher value of P_{MC}.

Notice two other ways to raise the P_{MC} beyond merely elevating the venous reservoir itself. First, you could add more blood to the system. This would raise the level within the reservoir and accomplish the same thing as lifting the whole reservoir. Second, you could shrink the size of the reservoir container while keeping the amount of blood constant. This would again raise the height of the blood column and elevate P_{MC}. Why mention these? The body does the same things, as we shall see later on.

Effect of Depressing Contractility

If we kept the level of the reservoir P_{MC} constant and instead caused the heart in some way to pump less efficiently, the P_{RA} would rise as right atrial inflow temporarily exceeded outflow. This increased P_{RA} would in turn depress venous return through the Ohm's law relation until a new steady state was reached, where again right atrial output would equal venous return, but at a lower level than previously. Graphically we would have moved from normal operating point A to point C along the same venous return curve. If the heart were to have stopped entirely, flow ($\dot{Q}_{in}$) would go to zero and P_{RA} would rise to P_{MC}. This situation is seen as point D in the figure, where the abscissa intercept takes the value P_{MC}. It should be evident that the P_{RA} intercept for each such curve will characterize the P_{MC} for that curve; that is, raising the reservoir height (P_{MC}) will move you to a new, higher venous return curve. The slope of each curve is $\dot{Q}/(P_{RA} - P_{MC})$, or the negative reciprocal of Rv (which is $(P_{MC} - P_{RA})/\dot{Q}$). Although Rv is probably also subject to change and regulation in intact animals, we will not allow it to change in the discussion that follows. We'll keep the slopes constant, even though the positions of the curves change.

Effect of Increasing Contractility

Instead of depressing the heart, it could have been stimulated with drugs, causing it to pump so well that it took P_{RA} down to atmospheric pressure ($P_{RA} = 0$). This would have decreased the back pressure across Rv and caused $\dot{Q}_{in}$ to increase with the creation of a new operating point E. Suppose the heart could pull P_{RA} below atmospheric pressure to negative levels. What would happen? Would $\dot{Q}_{in}$ increase still further? Probably not. At this point external pressure on the vena cava would exceed internal pressure, a negative transmural pressure would exist, and the veins would collapse, thus limiting $\dot{Q}_{in}$ essentially to the level it had achieved at $P_{RA} = 0$. This situation is illustrated by point F on the venous return curve which has a near zero slope in this region.

Why such a strange, complicated plot as Fig. 4.11 is used will be revealed in the next two sections, where cardiac output and its convivial relation to venous return are discussed.

The Hidden Pulmonary Circulation

Up to this point we have been discussing right atrial venous return and ignoring right ventricular and pulmonary circulation. In life, the systemic venular reservoir is the site of an effective P_{MC} with an Rv lying between it and the right atrium. In the Starling preparation the pulmonary venous reservoir is hidden from view, just as it is in life, yet it seems to function as does the artificial system created by Starling for input to the right side of the circulation, determining in the same way how much blood will flow into the left atrial/left ventricular complex. Pressures in the pulmonary veins and left atrium, however, tend to exceed those in comparable right-sided structures by a few mm Hg.

Cardiac Output versus Atrial Pressure: The Output Curve

Starling's Law of the Heart

Given an adequate input, what can the heart do on its own, unencumbered by reflexes and hormones? Starling found out. Using the heart–lung preparation he found that "the energy of contraction, however measured, is a function of the length of the muscle fibre," and "within physiological limits the larger the volume of the heart, the greater are the energy of its contraction and the amount of chemical change at each contraction." He came to this conclusion by studying what happened to stroke work when he changed venous return by elevating or lowering the venous reservoir, and what happened when he increased the resistance to left ventricular outflow, Ra (2).

Effect of Raising P_{MC}

Consider what happens when the venous reservoir (P_{MC}) is raised and, as we already know, venous return to the right atrium/right ventricle is increased. The heart at first continues to eject the same stroke volume. With the same flow out and more flow in, the ventricle will begin to swell as it accumulates blood. Instead of swelling and perhaps bursting, the heart automatically becomes capable of pumping out precisely what is delivered to it. The only significant changes are increases in end diastolic ventricular volume (EDV) and end diastolic ventricular pressure (EDP). This also means an increase in ventricular preload, calculated from the law of Laplace.

At this higher volume the heart will also be pumping against a higher arterial pressure than before, because a higher flow is being pushed through the arterial resistance downstream (Ohm's law). This means that ventricular afterload will also have increased.

A higher flow delivered against a higher pressure means more stroke work than before, and this ability to do more work as a result of increased ventricular stretch is called the Frank–Starling effect. There will also be an increased right atrial pressure, reflecting the higher end diastolic pressure necessarily stretching the ventricle until output matches input.

Starling found the relation of stroke work to end diastolic volume to be curvilinear (Fig. 4.12). Such a plot is often called a Starling curve, and variants of it are called ventricular function curves.

To reiterate, while the ventricle was temporarily being filled more rapidly than it could empty itself, it soon became stretched and thereby endowed with enough vigor (increased stroke work) to pump out as much as it received. When, on the other hand, the heart was supplied with less blood than before, it would shrink in size and adjust its stroke work and cardiac output downward appropriately.

Effect of Raising Circulatory Resistance

Otto Frank, toward the end of the last century, had done similar experiments with frog hearts, but instead of using increased input to stretch them, he accomplished the same thing by forcing them to work against a higher arteriolar-plus-capillary resistance (Ra in Fig. 4.9). He allowed venous return to continue unabated from a

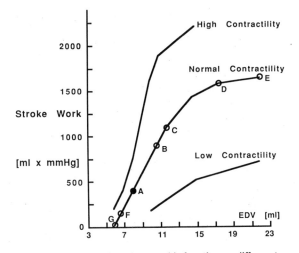

FIG. 4.12. Starling curves (stroke work) for three different contractilities at constant resistance.

large reservoir while the heart's normal force of contraction proved to be temporarily unable to generate the higher arterial pressures necessary to overcome this higher resistance. The result was that blood backed up in the heart, and the heart began to stretch. Frank found that the heart responded to this load by putting out more stroke work, with intermediate steps being increases in wall stress and end diastolic volume. Starling followed this lead and did comparable experiments in the dog heart–lung preparation. He found, as he had noted before with increased venous return, that the heart first stretched to a larger volume and thereby could do more stroke work.

Frank–Starling Curves Using Stroke Work
and End Diastolic Volume

Figure 4.12 shows curvilinear plots of the Frank–Starling relationship for a small imaginary dog heart and lung with a fixed arteriolar resistance. Stroke work is approximately equal to $\bar{P}a \times SV$, where $\bar{P}a$ is mean arterial pressure in mm Hg, and SV is stroke volume in ml. Stroke work is plotted against EDV in ml. This heart is assumed to operate near point A on the normal contractility curve with an EDV of 8 ml, a stroke work of 396 mm Hg × ml (corresponding to a stroke volume of 4 ml), and a mean arterial systolic pressure of 100 mm Hg. Heart rate is fixed at 150/min throughout. In response to an infusion of blood generated by raising the reservoir (increased P_{MC}), the system's operating point moves along the normal isocontractility curve to point B. This happens because the input of blood into the right atrium for a while is greater than the output, causing the EDV to increase. Because of this larger EDV the heart begins working harder and is soon able to put out what comes in. Note that this higher output must flow through the fixed arteriolar-plus-capillary resistance, Ra, and hence develops a higher aortic pressure, Pa, because the distal end of Ra has a fixed pressure of zero in the heart–lung preparation.

Two other curves are included in Fig. 4.12. The one labeled low contractility shows how the heart might perform under the influence of depressing drugs such as barbiturates or following a myocardial infarction. The major finding should be clear: At a given stretch (P_{RA}) less stroke work is available when contractility is low. This new Starling curve is therefore an isocontractility line representing a new, less-healthy state of the myocardium. We have also included an analogous curve for a high contractility state of the myocardium. We could have reached this curve by an intravenous infusion of epinephrine or norepinephrine. On this new Starling curve, in a new isocontractility state, the heart is capable of performing higher work per stroke for a given amount of stretch.

Other Derived Curves

Data from curves in Fig. 4.12 will be used to derive still other circulatory relationships. These are discussed in the sections immediately following.

Frank–Starling Curves Using Cardiac Output and P_{RA}

In an attempt to relate inflow more readily to outflow and to unify our understanding of how the circulation works, Arthur Guyton and hi̇ ᷉ollaborators chose to transform this classical Starling curve a bit, piotting cardiac output (instead of stroke work) versus atrial pressure. The reasoning went something like this: Mean right atrial pressure is practically identical to right ventricular end diastolic pressure, which in turn is closely related to ventricular end diastolic volume, Starling's variable. This latter relationship changes as ventricular compliance changes but will be reasonably fixed if not linear over a wide range of physiological conditions. Right atrial pressure, on the other hand, also appears as a variable in the venous return relationship, so we are now given the possibility of plotting both cardiac input and cardiac output on the same graph versus right atrial pressure.

The same data used for normal contractility in Fig. 4.12 have been replotted as cardiac output versus right atrial pressure at constant resistance (R) in Fig. 4.13. It should be emphasized that in both plots we held total peripheral resistance (Ra + Rv) constant while we changed venous return by varying P_{MC}. We made another important model assumption in going from Fig. 4.12 to Fig. 4.13: We used the real-life situation of ending the resistance Ra with pressure P_{MC}, instead of pressure equal to zero as occurs in the true Starling heart–lung preparation. This will cause calculated cardiac outputs to differ by perhaps 5–10% between these models, but

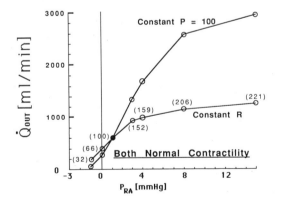

FIG. 4.13. Starling curve (cardiac output) with resistance or pressure held constant.

at the same time, it makes the calculations easier and the model more physiologic.

Fixed Resistance versus Fixed Arterial Pressure

The points in Figs. 4.13 and 4.14 correspond to the same points on the labeled curve in Fig. 4.12. In Fig. 4.13 the plot of flow versus atrial pressure **at constant peripheral resistance** (Ra + Rv) shows that cardiac output plateaus earlier than stroke work does in the more conventional Starling diagram. The reason that flow doesn't increase as rapidly as stroke work does is that more and more work must be expended in creating higher pressures at high flows. These pressures have been indicated beside each point as values in parentheses. (For ease of calculation we have equated mean systolic arterial pressure with mean arterial pressure.) We have illustrated this idea in another way in the same figure by showing what the heart should be able to do if we had held arterial pressure fixed at 100 mm Hg by lowering Ra appropriately as we increased venous return and ultimately P_{RA}. The constant pressure curve is the result. A given amount of work can represent high flows at normal pressure or much lower flows at high pressures. Fig. 4.13 illustrates both the high cost one pays for elevated blood

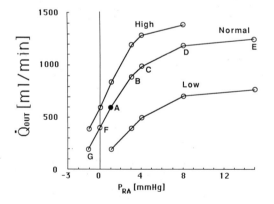

FIG. 4.14. Starling curves (cardiac output) for three different contractilities.

pressures and the pivotal role arteriolar resistance probably plays in controlling blood pressure.

A Family of Starling Curves

In Fig. 4.14 we replot the Starling curves from Fig. 4.12 for all three contractilities, now using cardiac output ($\dot{Q}$) as the ordinate. To reemphasize: all three curves have been calculated for fixed peripheral arteriolar, capillary, and venous resistances (constant R) from data in Fig. 4.12 and from the definitions of minute work and circulatory resistance. P_{MC} is the true independent variable, and P_{RA}, Pa, and $\dot{Q}$ are all determined from it.

Arterial Pressure versus Right Atrial Pressure

To get a better feeling for how the heart might perform if Ra and Rv were held constant, have a look at Fig. 4.15, in which we've used the data from Fig. 4.12 to calculate the mean systolic arterial pressures attained at each P_{RA}. Considering that mean arterial pressure in humans is normally around $\overline{95}$, with a mean arterial pressure during systole perhaps 10 mm Hg higher, the heart in these figures is wasting a lot of energy by raising pressures above

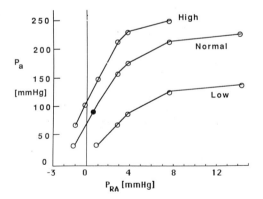

FIG. 4.15. Mean arterial pressure; resistance held constant for three different contractilities.

this level. Of course, if you had hypertension with a relatively fixed, high Ra you would probably be glad your heart was equal to the task. Although Fig. 4.15 appears to indicate the contrary, Pa is not a good index of contractility because it is strongly regulated by reflex control mechanisms in the intact animal. In the absence of such controls (i.e., heart rate, Ra and Rv are held constant here), Fig. 4.15 shows how Pa in the isolated heart will respond to changes in P_{RA}.

Ejection Fraction versus P_{MC}

Remember that high ejection fraction is sometimes used as an indication of high heart contractility. How does ejection fraction behave when contractility is held constant but P_{MC} is changed? If it is a good index, it should stay constant. The results of our model calculations are shown in Fig. 4.16. Here we have assumed that EDV in this dog can be given by the very arbitrary formula: EDV (ml)= P_{RA} + 7. We have then calculated SV by dividing cardiac outputs by the fixed heart rate of 150/min, and further determined ejection fraction as SV/EDV. The exact shapes of these curves are highly dependent upon our arbitrary and perhaps unphysiological choice of a formula to estimate EDV, but the general notion presented

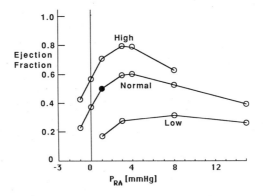

FIG. 4.16. Ejection fraction for three different contractilities.

is still true: At a given EDV (stretch) higher contractility will generally be associated with a higher ejection fraction. The fall off of
ejection fraction at higher P_{RA} is real because the heart is putting
more energy into raising pressure and less energy into raising cardiac
output.

Effects of Changing System Variables

Change P_{MC} but Keep Contractility Constant

Figure 4.17 combines the cardiac input curves (Fig. 4.11) with
the cardiac output curves (Fig. 4.14), both of which have P_{RA} as
common abscissas. The idea behind this is that in the steady state
cardiac input and cardiac output must be equal (and of course
P_{RA} is equal to itself) so that the heart will be operating at the
crossing point of an input curve with an output curve. Starting
with point A as our normal operating point, we now see that we
can move upward to point 1 on the normal contractility curve by
increasing P_{MC}. In the intact animal this could be achieved by an
increase in venous tone or an increase in (venous) blood volume.
This latter might be produced by a transfusion or a transfer of

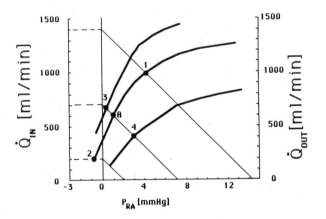

FIG. 4.17. A combined input/output plot.

tissue fluid into the vascular compartment. We could also have moved in the opposite direction to point 2 on the same isocontractility curve by bleeding the dog or otherwise depleting its blood volume and thus lowering P_{MC}. By moving along this curve we have affected cardiac function through the stretch mechanism, but we have not altered the heart's basic contractility. The circulatory system has been markedly expanded or contracted in the process however (a 10–15% volume change).

Change Contractility but Keep P_{MC} Constant

Point 3 can be reached by an increase in heart contractility with no change in P_{MC} and probably little change in total blood volume. This could be achieved by the infusion of an agent like epinephrine. We can move to point 4 merely by depressing the myocardium with an anesthetic agent. In both these cases we are dealing with changes along a venous return curve where P_{MC} is essentially constant. Having reached point 4, changes in P_{MC} will then take us along the low contractility curve in either direction to new operating points.

A caveat: The output curves used in Fig. 4.17 were all obtained using the assumption of constant arteriolar-plus-capillary resistance, Ra. This situation is appropriate for the Starling heart–lung preparation and for animals whose circulatory reflexes have been purposely paralyzed. A more physiologic picture would have resulted had we superimposed the input curves on a set of cardiac output curves similar to the steeper, constant pressure curve of Fig. 4.13 (upper curve). In the intact animal changes in pressure are quickly buffered by the baroreceptor mechanism so that arterial pressure is regulated by changing both arteriolar resistance and heart contractility (and also heart rate and probably venous tone). Perhaps you can see why Starling wanted to study the isolated heart and lung without these complications. You should conclude from all this that the only way to move the operating point is to move one of the curves.

Remembrance of Things Past

This is probably a good place to repeat what was presented in Chapter 1. There are four main, short-term control mechanisms operating in the circulation:

1. Heart rate
2. Heart contractility
3. Arteriolar resistance (Ra, neglecting capillary resistance)
4. Venous tone (determining P_{MC})

You should now have a better appreciation of the primacy of these parameters and of the secondary nature of:

1. Cardiac output ($\dot{Q}$)
2. Arterial pressure (Pa)
3. Atrial pressure (P_{RA})

Arterial pressure and flow, both from this latter group, are being maintained by the body. It uses the four control mechanisms (plus others) to do its job.

Summary

Increased contractility is indicated by an increased ejection fraction and usually is associated with lower values of both P_{RA} and EDV for comparable cardiac outputs. **Decreased contractility** is associated with the opposite findings. A greatly increased EDV, for example, is the hallmark of cardiac failure. **The Starling mechanism** is invoked by ventricular stretch. Stretch in turn is dependent upon P_{MC} and upon heart contractility as is seen in Fig. 4.17.

A cautionary note: We have not taken the data for the figures in this section from real animals, yet we have pushed their interpretation quite far. To push anymore is to find inconsistencies; the model will surely break down at some point. In the intact animal the high pressures we have calculated are rarely allowed to occur and are rapidly corrected by reflex mechanisms that we shall discuss in more detail later.

INTRINSIC PERFORMANCE *IN VIVO:* VENTRICULAR FUNCTION CURVES AND OTHER MATTERS

Introduction

This section deals with more Starling curves, not those derived from the heart–lung preparation, but curves from studies of whole animals, even people. In this setting they are called ventricular function curves. As in the heart–lung preparation, we have made an attempt to keep heart rate and contractility, as well as circulatory resistances and compliances, all constant. Because contractility is difficult even to define, the concept of holding such a thing constant is probably unrealistic. Nonetheless, we shall proceed.

The aim in these laboratory and clinical studies is the same: to find out what the heart can do by itself. In the clinical situation the cardiologist might be asking whether a patient's heart muscle has been damaged by coronary artery disease or whether his signs and symptoms are due to valve malfunctions. The results could suggest the need for coronary artery replacement instead of valve replacement, for example.

In People

In the usual clinical setting it is impossible to obtain enough data to inscribe a complete left ventricular stroke work versus EDV curve. Instead, the values obtained are compared with normal figures for a patient of comparable age, sex, height, and weight, and the findings evaluated along with all other data to come to a conclusion.

In Animals

In experimental studies in animals, one is in a position to intervene more drastically and get ventricular function curves which mimic the heart–lung data more closely. Such curves should look like Fig. 4.12, that is, interventions that improve myocardial function (increase contractility) should result in the ability to perform more stroke work at a given value of ventricular stretch. Maintaining contractility and circulatory variables constant along each curve is the hard part. The experiments will usually have been done to demonstrate that certain drugs either increase or decrease ventricular function (contractility). In assessing the results, one should be aware that drug interventions can seriously alter such circulatory variables as heart rate, arteriolar and venous resistance, venous tone, and arterial compliance. Note also that the gambits used to vary EDV (for example, blood transfusion and bleeding) may well alter these same variables. Because these variables are supposed to stay constant while ventricular function experiments are performed, you should look for substantiating evidence in such studies.

Passive Properties of the Heart

What about the passive properties of ventricles, atria, and the pericardium? Are they important for heart function? More and more evidence suggests that they are, and this is a current area of cardiac research.

The Pericardium

Consider first the pericardium. It's floppy up to a point, and then it's very hard to stretch it more. There are diseases (viral and tubercular, for example) producing a constrictive pericarditis in which reasonably normal ventricles cannot fill to normal volumes simply because the pericardial sac has become too small. Recent laboratory findings suggest that even in normal animals (including people), the pericardium may limit the degree to which a ventricle can be filled. There is also evidence that overfilling one ventricle may prevent the adequate filling of its neighbor because they occupy the same sac. In the light of these findings, experiments done with the pericardium removed have probably been less physiological than those in which it has remained intact.

Intrathoracic Pressure

While we're dealing with the effect of ventricular neighbors on ventricular function, what about the influence of the pressure in the intrathoracic cavity that surrounds the pericardium? Does it affect ventricular function? It does. The pleural pressure at end-expiration is about -5 cm H_2O, that is, 5 cm H_2O **below** atmospheric pressure. This keeps the lungs from collapsing, and it also pulls on the pericardium and ventricles from the outside. When you take a deep breath this pressure becomes even more negative, sucking air into the alveoli, but also sucking blood into vascular areas within the thorax from systemic veins. This negative pressure surrounding the heart helps explain why average atrial pressures are near zero or even negative (with respect to atmospheric pressure).

Ventricular Compliance

The compliance (stretchability) of ventricular muscle is also capable of altering apparent ventricular function. Just as a given preload will stretch a muscle strip to different lengths depending on the muscle's inherent stiffness (opposite of stretchability), so a given end diastolic pressure will produce different end diastolic volumes depending on ventricular compliance. The more compliant (floppy) the ventricle, the easier it will be stretched and the higher the volume at a given pressure. Therefore, because ventricular compliance is not the same in all animals, end diastolic pressure is not a perfect indicator of end diastolic volume (ventricular stretch). Ventricular compliance may not only differ from heart to heart, but it may even change over time in the same heart. Diseases can both stiffen and loosen our myocardial fibers, affecting cardiac function independently of inherent contractility changes. Even within a single cardiac cycle, hearts are more compliant at low volumes than when they are overstretched, and their calculated stretchability may vary depending on the state of contraction.

Summary

The attempt to quantitate something called contractility in the intact animal has not been overwhelmingly successful. Investigators continue to look for indices of inherent muscle performance, however, because clinical therapy depends critically on the state of the heart. The indices we have at present: *dP/dt*, V_{max}, ejection fraction, slope of the ventricular pressure-volume curve, etc., while not perfect, are useful; and we should seriously try to understand their physiologic importance and limitations.

EXTRINSIC REGULATION OF CARDIAC FUNCTION

Introduction

The Frank–Starling effect exemplifies the inherent properties of heart muscle and how well the heart can regulate itself. Contractility, however, was thought to be independent of the Frank–Starling effect. The following section deals with the regulation of cardiac muscle properties by extrinsic means.

Contractility

The sympathetics are sympathetic to contractility. The vagus is quite vague about it. This is another way of saying that there is little evidence for physiologic control of contractility by the vagus (or its messenger, acetylcholine). Ventricular muscle is heavily laden with sympathetic nerve endings containing norepinephrine. Norepinephrine increases contractility. Stimulating sympathetics increases contractility and depletes myocardial norepinephrine stores. Ergo, the sympathetics regulate contractility. There even seems to be a baseline activity within this system, so that lowered contractility will result if the sympathetics are shut off.

The released norepinephrine has only to reach nearby beta$_1$ receptors on muscle cell membranes to elicit this effect, but the availability of such receptors raises the possibility that other potential beta$_1$

agonists such as circulating epinephrine can also alter contractility. In general, however, such blood-borne or humoral regulation of contractility is not considered important in most physiological situations, even though administration of similar compounds as drugs can produce drastic changes in contractility.

Within muscle cells the effect of norepinephrine is probably mediated by increased Ca^{2+} levels. New evidence says that even the Frank–Starling stretch effect is mediated by increased Ca^{2+} influx into muscle cells, so Starling and contractility may have one common final action at the Ca^{2+} level in causing increased force development. The two paths to increased Ca^{2+} levels still represent two important and basically **different** physiologic means of force development, however.

Drugs that deplete catecholamine stores (norepinephrine is a catecholamine) in heart muscle, or that block beta$_1$ receptors, can therefore cause potential decreases in contractility, even to the point of producing cardiac failure or arterial hypotension. This side effect is an important one for a number of recently introduced drugs.

Heart Rate

The other major handle the body has on cardiac function is heart rate. It is controlled by continuous vagal and sympathetic discharges, with vagal influence predominating in the resting state. It is as if we were driving with one foot pushing on the sympathetic accelerator while the other pressed even more firmly on the vagal brake. To slow down the rate, just increase the vagus and decrease the sympathetics. To speed up the rate, just back off on the vagus and increase the sympathetics.

This action all takes place within the SA node through mechanisms described in Chapter 2. Again, cell receptors of the beta$_1$ type are involved in sympathetic action, and acetylcholine receptors mediate the vagal response. Humoral influences are not thought to regulate function here in normal physiologic states. Drugs can change the heart rate in the same way they can influence contractility, by modifying the release, recovery, and reception of transmitters.

When considering the effect of a pure increase in heart rate on cardiac output, the natural tendency is to think: double the rate, double the output. Careful, it's not that simple. The hand-operated pump on a farm probably works that way because its input pressure stays reasonably constant and keeps stroke volumes reasonably constant also. Not so the left ventricle! When the ventricle pumps faster and increases the output even a little bit, it concurrently "pumps down" the pressure in the adjoining atrium and leaves itself with less filling pressure. Output can't be greater than input and cardiac **input** is often limited.

Yet another way of looking at this is: Transient increases in output due to increases in heart rate may elevate arterial pressure (Pa) slightly, but they have little effect on the pressure within the large circulatory reservoir (P_{MC}). To the extent, though, that atrial pressure (P_{LA}, P_{RA}) is lowered, cardiac input will also increase somewhat because $\dot{Q}_{in} = (P_{MC} - P_{RA})/R_V$. Do not look for a simple doubling of output with a doubling of heart rate; cardiac input must also increase in some other way if one is to achieve a significant steady-state increase in cardiac output.

There is another important limitation on cardiac output as heart rate is increased above, say, 160–180 beats/min, and this also has to do with cardiac input. There is not enough time in diastole, when the rate is this fast, to get a stroke volume's worth of blood into the heart. This difficulty is compounded by the fact that faster rates are achieved by shortening diastole more than systole. When you encroach upon the rapid filling phase of diastole at heart rates above 180 or so, you are going to have **lower** outputs instead of higher ones. Athletes are subject to the same limitations as we nonathletes are; yet their maximal heart rates are only slightly higher. However, they start at lower resting rates than we do. Endurance athletes thus commonly have resting heart rates in the 30s, giving them a potential 5-fold increase in output, whereas we 72 beats/ min folk must be content with a mere 2½-fold change. Because these athletes' basal requirements for cardiac output are similar to ours, their stroke volumes at rest will have to be double ours, and their hearts will probably be larger as well.

Other Extrinsic Controls

While heart rate and contractility are considered the principal means by which we control our hearts, there are other possibilities, and these are the subject of continuing investigation.

For example, we now realize that the passive properties of the myocardium, such as its compliance and its plasticity, are important for adequate function. These variables do not hold still under different levels of sympathetic stimulation, and they may well help to regulate the circulation. The coronary arterial circulation seems from many studies to be unresponsive to known external control mechanisms in normal physiological states; yet there is continuing evidence that newly discovered agents (the prostaglandins, for example) and other agents (like norepinephrine) may have some effect. For example, a syndrome known as Prinzmetal's angina is associated with spasm of the coronary arterial tree, and this in turn may be related to release of some of the above agents. Because a muscle's function will be dependent upon its blood supply, this area of research will continue to be important for those interested in function and control.

We should point out that even the Frank–Starling mechanism itself might be subject to external control. At the level of this introductory text, we should continue to think of the length–tension mechanism as an inherent property of the heart. But allow the possibility that researchers will one day find that it has been controlled all along with agent X, to be available soon from your local pharmacy (by prescription only).

CARDIAC RESPONSES TO SIMPLE STRESSES IN THE ABSENCE OF EXTERNAL CONTROLS

Introduction

This section continues to deal with a stripped-down system isolated from many important circulatory consequences that we will consider in later sections.

In this analysis we have to answer the question: What repertoire of basic responses does the heart have? We will consider three of these: (1) the Frank–Starling effect, (2) contractility, and (3) heart rate.

We should also ask: What are the important stresses to which the heart is subject? It is frequently confronted by increases in venous return which require that it come up with higher outputs or burst. It frequently has to pump against a higher arteriolar resistance and thus has to generate higher pressures. We will also have to consider what happens when sympathetics and/or the vagus are stimulated, or when hormones mimicking these stimulations reach the heart via the bloodstream.

Response to Increased Venous Return

Let's deal first with an increase in cardiac input. This might have arisen because of an increase in venous tone, because a transfusion had been given, or even because the subject had gone from the standing to the lying position. If the output initially is unchanged, the increased input stretches the heart and clearly involves the Frank–Starling mechanism. It's important to remember that this is not a change in contractility.

To follow the changes, consider Fig. 4.17. Starting at normal operating point A, the increased $\dot{Q}_{in}$ will move the heart upward along the constant normal contractility line toward a new operating point 1. It will find itself on a new venous return curve, and hence a new, higher value of P_{MC} (now 14 mm Hg).

We've also increased P_{RA} from 1 to 4 mm Hg, which should tend to **impede** venous return. Does P_{MC} or P_{RA} win out? Assume that venous resistance stays constant in this analysis. The initial pressure gradient causing cardiac input was $P_{MC} - P_{RA} = 7 - 1 = 6$ mm Hg. In the new state $P_{MC} - P_{RA} = 14 - 4 = 10$ mm Hg, so flow will have increased.

What goes in, goes out, so in the steady state cardiac output will come to match input. This happens automatically on the graph, where the right-hand scale is the same as the left-hand scale.

What happens to Pa? If Rv, Ra (arteriolar-plus-capillary resistance), and heart rate are unchanged, and P_{RA} increases only slightly, the increase in $\dot{Q}_{out}$ will produce an increase in Pa, as can be seen from the Ohm's law relationship: $\bar{P}a - \bar{P}_{RA} = (Rv + Ra)\dot{Q}$.

The heart thus has increased its **stroke work** for two reasons: (1) it's working against a higher pressure, and (2) it's delivering a larger stroke volume. (Remember that stroke work = stroke volume × mean systolic arterial pressure.)

Because both P_{MC} (i.e., venular P) and Pa are higher, you can expect that capillary pressure intermediate between these two will also have risen.

Keep in mind that this analysis covers only **part** of the story. We have deliberately ignored such things as baroreceptors, contractility, and heart rate, all of which would have been changing drastically in real life.

Response to Increased Arteriolar Resistance

On Fig. 4.17, go back to the normal operating point A and consider what would happen if the arteriolar resistance were raised while contractility was kept constant. Certainly in the new steady state you would not expect a **higher** cardiac output. Tracing the effects of increased arteriolar resistance around the circulation isn't easy, however. Even for a computer it takes several iterations (repeated calculating trips) through the variables involved before the results settle down.

Consider as a first approximation that $\bar{P}_{MC}$ changes very little at first. After all, it is the pressure in a large, very compliant reservoir, and relatively large volume changes will be required to change it. Consider also that cardiac input on the other side of the heart from Ra will not be affected much at first. What is the result? $\bar{P}a - \bar{P}_{MC} = Ra\,\dot{Q}_{out}$ and the Frank–Starling effect ($\dot{Q}_{in} = \dot{Q}_{out}$) together indicate that a rise in Ra will produce an increase in mean arterial pressure, $\bar{P}a$.

How did the Frank–Starling effect get invoked? Continued input in the face of **transiently** decreased output stretched the heart and enabled it to produce more stroke work. This had to mean increased P_{RA}, which in turn tended to decrease cardiac input (from $P_{MC} - P_{RA} = Rv \times \dot{Q}_{in}$). Thus, in the new steady state $\dot{Q}_{in}$ and hence $\dot{Q}_{out}$ will both have fallen slightly.

We therefore have decreased $\dot{Q}_{in}$ and $\dot{Q}_{out}$ and increased P_{RA}. How can this fit in with Fig. 4.17? You've got to draw a **new curve, below** the normal contractility curve and more or less parallel to it. It will look like a curve for slightly lower contractility (but it really is not). The new operating point will be at the intersection of this new curve with the original venous return curve: to the right and downward from operating point A and heading toward point 4. The heart still operates on the same venous return curve because P_{MC} has not changed. On Fig. 4.17 it becomes evident that a higher Ra makes the heart perform as if it had a lower contractility. It must work harder (higher $\bar{P}a$) to keep cardiac output up (but it isn't quite succeeding). This is where people with essential hypertension find themselves; they're obviously in trouble.

Response to Sympathetic or Parasympathetic Stimulation of the Heart

Suppose we held Ra and P_{MC} constant (not easy) and stimulated (one at a time) each division of the motor nervous supply to the heart. What would happen?

Sympathetic Stimulation

Stimulating the cardiac sympathetics will release norepinephrine within the ventricular muscle and in the atrial wall near the SA and AV nodes. Try to predict the results. You're right if you said that both ventricular contractility and heart rate will rise.

Let's consider the effect of **increased contractility** first. On Fig. 4.17 we'll be starting at point A and going up the venous return curve to the left toward point 3. We're still on this same venous return curve because we haven't done anything that would change P_{MC}. The increased pumping ability of the heart has not only raised cardiac output, it has also pumped down the pressure in its immediate reservoirs, the atria, so P_{RA} becomes lower in the process.

For a steady state to exist $\dot{Q}_{in}$ has to rise to equal $\dot{Q}_{out}$. How could this happen? The secret lies in lowered P_{RA}, because $\dot{Q}_{in} = (P_{MC} - P_{RA})/Rv$, and we haven't purposely changed P_{MC} or Rv. Note that decreased P_{RA} will mean less stretch of the ventricle at end diastole and therefore less Frank–Starling effect. The heart thus has sacrificed some force development by one mechanism in gaining more by another.

What about the **increased heart rate** that comes along with sympathetic stimulation? Let's consider the effect of a rise in heart rate alone. **If** stroke volume were somehow kept the same, then doubling the heart rate should double the cardiac output. The **if** is too big, however, and this doesn't happen. **If,** on the other hand, cardiac input were left unchanged, then a doubling of heart rate couldn't raise the output at all. The heart would merely be operating with a doubled rate and a halved stroke volume. Again, this extreme **if** of the opposite kind doesn't happen. The truth lies somewhere in between, and things probably happen in the following way:

An increase in rate will certainly begin to increase cardiac output, but ventricular EDV and P_{RA} will drop as the heart is pumped dry. By now you must realize that the decreasing P_{RA} will also cause an increase in venous return. This increase still won't be proportional to the increase in heart rate, although it will allow $\dot{Q}_{out}$ to rise somewhat. Limiting cardiac function will be the fact that EDV is smaller, producing a consequently smaller Frank–Starling effect: a lowered force of contraction. None of this is demonstrable on Fig. 4.17 because this diagram was generated by a heart with a fixed rate.

The combination of increased contractility and increased rate will tend to raise output more than either alone. However, the heart will still be limited by the venous return available, and venous return will not increase further as P_{RA} is taken below about 0 mm Hg. The only way to make efficient use of increased rate and contractility is to have P_{MC} increase as well. More on this later.

Parasympathetic Stimulation

For completeness, stimulation of cardiac vagal efferents needs to be mentioned. The effect will be primarily on the SA node with a production of a slower heart rate. The overall effects are the opposite of those with increased rate above: a decreased cardiac output and input. Input is decreased because less frequent emptying allows EDV and P_{RA} to rise, impeding venous return. The increased stretch will also invoke the Frank–Starling effect, however, and tend to oppose these changes by increasing the force of contraction somewhat. There seems to be little if any **direct** vagal effect on contractility.

SUMMARY

This section has been a long one because mechanics of the heart is a complex topic. We have oversimplified our presentation through the use of streamlined models. The area is still being actively investigated, and one can expect even these simplified explanations to be somewhat out of date in a couple of years.

This section introduced the concepts of **preload, afterload,** and **contractility** from experiments dealing with linear muscle strips applied in the analysis of ventricular function. You should have begun to understand how variables such as initial muscle length and maximum shortening velocity (V_{max}) are useful in describing both the linear and ventricular systems.

The events of the cardiac cycle were described in some detail, first as temporal plots of selected variables and then as pressure–volume plots. We related electrical to mechanical events and showed how the intrinsic cardiac events affected the variables one could conveniently measure.

We then considered the Starling heart–lung preparation, a model system representing the heart unaffected by outside control mechanisms. We described in detail how this system responded to changes in input flow, output resistance, heart rate, and contractility. In the process you should have grasped what the primary and secondary

circulatory variables are, and just how they might change when
the system is perturbed.

REFERENCES

1. Wiggers, C.J. *Physiology in Health and Disease.* Philadelphia: Lea & Febiger,
   1954.
2. *Starling's Linacre lecture given in 1915,* London: Longmans, Green, and Co.,
   1981.

QUESTIONS

Use curves 1–6 in Fig. 4.18 to answer **Questions 4.01–4.04.**

4.01. A person whose resting $\dot{V}_{O_2}$ was 300 ml/min, STPD, whose
arterial O_2 content was 200 ml O_2/L blood, and whose mixed
venous O_2 content was 150 ml O_2/L blood would be operating
at the intersection of curves:

a. 1 and 4   d. 2 and 4
b. 1 and 5   e. 2 and 5
c. 1 and 6

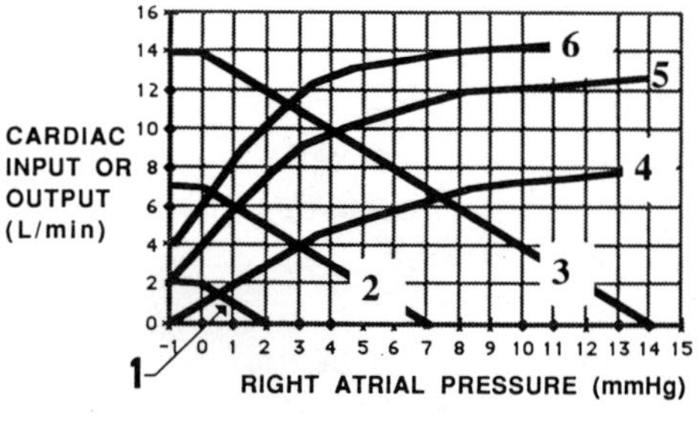

FIG. 4.18.   See Questions 4.01–4.04.

4.02. A person having a mean circulatory pressure of 7 mm Hg, a mean arterial pressure of 93 mm Hg, and a peripheral resistance of 22.5 mm Hg/(L/min) would be operating at the intersection of curves:

a. 1 and 4
b. 1 and 5
c. 1 and 6
d. 2 and 4
e. 2 and 5

4.03. Shifting from an operating point at the intersection of curves 2 and 5 to an operating point at the intersection of curves 3 and 6 would be best explained by:

a. Acute hemorrhage.
b. Acute fluid overload.
c. Cardiac failure.
d. Moderate exercise.
e. Administration of a drug whose only effect was to raise contractility.

4.04. If a person whose normal operating point is at the intersection of curves 2 and 5 were to change to an operating point at the intersection of curves 2 and 4, this might best be explained by:

a. Acute hemorrhage.
b. Acute fluid overload.
c. Cardiac failure.
d. Moderate exercise.
e. Administration of a drug whose only effect was to raise contractility.

Use curves 1–6 in Fig. 4.19 to answer **Questions 4.05–4.08.**

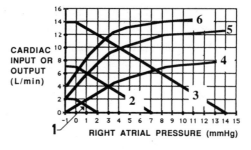

FIG. 4.19. See Questions 4.05–4.08.

4.05. Suppose a normal person has a P_{MC} = 14 mm Hg, $\dot{V}_{O_2}$ = 880 ml/min, STPD, arterial O_2 content of 200 ml/L, and right ventricular O_2 content of 120 ml/L. This person's right atrial pressure in mm Hg would be closest to:

a. −1   d. 4
b. 1   e. 7
c. 3

4.06. If the person described in Question 4.05 had a mean arterial pressure of 95 mm Hg, his venous resistance would be closest to which following fraction of total peripheral resistance?

a. 0.050   d. 0.120
b. 0.056   e. 0.200
c. 0.116

4.07. Suppose a different person whose cardiovascular system was operating in a steady state at the intersections of curves 2 and 5 were given an infusion of 1,000 ml of blood. If his cardiovascular system now operates at the intersection of curves 3 and 5, his venous compliance in ml/mm Hg would be closest to:

a. 71   d. 500
b. 143   e. 1,000
c. 333

4.08. A person's cardiovascular system is operating at the intersection of curves 3 and 6 in a steady state. A coronary occlusion (heart attack), immediately causing ventricular fibrillation, would cause his right atrial pressure within seconds to:

a. Fall by about 4 mm Hg.
b. Become atmospheric as veins collapse.
c. Rise by about 1 mm Hg.
d. Rise by about 4 mm Hg.
e. Rise by about 11 mm Hg.

Figure 4.20 shows the pressure–volume relationship of the left ventricle of a patient in a steady state. The oxygen uptake measured with a spirometer is 300 ml/min, STPD, and heart rate is 75/min. Use the pressure–volume curve in Fig. 4.20 to answer **Questions 4.09–4.12.**

4.09. Which of the points (A–E) corresponds most closely in time with the peak of the "v" wave in the jugular venous pulse?

4.10. Which of the points (A–E) corresponds most closely in time with the "a" wave of the jugular venous pulse?

4.11. Which of the points (A–E) corresponds most closely in time with the second heart sound?

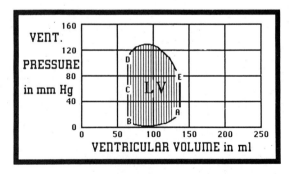

FIG. 4.20. See Questions 4.09–4.12.

4.12. Which of the points (A–E) corresponds most closely in time with the point at which aortic pressure reaches its diastolic value?

The wall thickness of an essentially spherical left ventricle can be considered constant at 1.5 cm throughout the cardiac cycle. Measured transmural ventricular pressures are: 15 mm Hg as the mitral valve opens, 20 mm Hg as the mitral valve closes, 70 mm Hg as the aortic valve opens, 85 mm Hg as the aortic valve closes, and maximally, 100 mm Hg when 0.8 of the stroke volume (SV) has been ejected. Suppose that the ventricular end diastolic volume (EDV) is 268 ml and the cardiac output is 4.5 L/min at a heart rate (HR) of 90/min. Use these data to answer **Questions 4.13–4.15.**

4.13. The left ventricular ejection fraction is closest to:

a. 0.1   d. 0.4
b. 0.2   e. 0.5
c. 0.3

4.14. The left ventricular preload in mm Hg is closest to:

a. 15   d. 34
b. 20   e. 43
c. 27

4.15. Maximum afterload calculable from the above data in mm Hg is closest to:

a. 85   d. 126
b. 93   e. 186
c. 100

Use the curves in Fig. 4.21, which could have been obtained from a dog heart–lung preparation, to answer **Questions 4.16 and 4.17.**

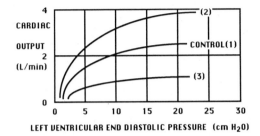

FIG. 4.21. See Questions 4.16 and 4.17.

4.16. Curve 2 might differ from control for any of the following reasons EXCEPT:

a. Stimulation of the stellate ganglion.
b. Stimulation of vagal efferent nerves to the heart.
c. Infusion of norepinephrine.
d. Increased myocardial contractility.
e. Increased firing in postganglionic sympathetic nerves to the heart.

4.17. Curve 3 might differ from the control because of:

a. Increased venous return.
b. Increased oxygen concentration in inspired air.
c. Administration of atropine, which blocks action of the vagus nerve.
d. Cardiac failure.
e. Administration of epinephrine.

ANSWERS

4.01. e. Use the Fick principle to determine that $\dot{Q}$ = 6 L/min. Curves 2 and 5 are the only ones that intersect at that $\dot{Q}$.

4.02. d. The P_{MC} = 7 mm Hg defines curve 2 as the venous filling curve for this person. Use Ohm's law to determine which intersection with curve 2 (and therefore which $\dot{Q}$ and P_{RA}) will fill the bill here. The intersection of curve 2 with curve 4 yields a $\dot{Q}$ = 4 L/min and a P_{RA} = 3 mm Hg. Testing the values with Ohm's law yields: $\dot{Q}$ = $P_{driving}/R$; 4 L/min = (93 − 3) mm Hg/ [22.5 mm Hg/(L/min)].

4.03. d. The only one of the choices which is consistent with shifts to a higher filling curve AND to a higher contractility curve is exercise.

4.04. c. The only one of the choices which is consistent with a shift to a lower contractility curve is cardiac failure.

4.05. c. The P_{MC} of 14 mm Hg defines curve 3 as the filling curve. Using the Fick principle to calculate that $\dot{Q}$ = 11 L/min identifies the intersection of curves 3 and 6 as the operating point, and approximately 3 mm Hg as the P_{RA}.

4.06. d. The total peripheral resistance, R, = $P_{driving}/\dot{Q}$ = (95 − 3) mm Hg/(11 L/min) = 8.36. The venous resistance is defined by the $P_{driving}$ from the beginning to the end of the veins divided by the $\dot{Q}$. R = $(P_{MC} - P_{RA})/\dot{Q}$ = (14 − 3) mm Hg/(11 L/min) = 1 mm Hg/(L/min). The slope of the venous filling curve gives this information also. 1/8.36 = 0.1196.

4.07. b. The 1000 ml of blood will go mostly to the veins, where it has caused the P_{MC} to increase by 7 mm Hg.
C = $\Delta V/\Delta P$ = 1000 ml/7 mm Hg = 143 ml/mm Hg.

4.08. e. The P_{RA} and all other pressures will move towards the P_{MC}.

4.09. Point B. The upstroke of the "v" wave (reflecting the gradual rise in the atrial pressure) is caused by blood "damming up" as venous return continues into the atria while the atrioventricular valves are closed. The pressure suddenly falls (downstroke of the "v" wave) as the atrioventricular valves open and allow the ventricles to begin filling. Filling of the ventricles begins at point B.

4.10. Point A. The "a" wave of the venous pulse results from atrial contraction, which occurs near the end of ventricular filling. Ventricular filling ends at point A.

4.11. Point D. The second heart sound is caused by the closure of the aortic and pulmonic valves, at the very end of systolic ejection.

4.12. Point E. The onset of systolic ejection prevents the aortic pressure from falling further.

4.13. b. $\dot{Q}$ = HR × SV; SV = (4500 ml/min)/90 beats/min = 50 ml/beat. Ejection fraction = SV/EDV = 50/268 = 0.19.

4.14. c. Load on a spherical ventricle (its wall stress) at any given point in its cycle is defined by Laplace's law for a sphere, where wall stress = S = $(P_{TM} \times r)/2h$. The point in the cycle at which one would calculate preload is just at the end of ventricular filling, or just at the closure of the atrioventricular valves. At this point, ventricular pressure = 20 mm Hg and the ventricle contains its EDV, given here = 268 ml. Volume of a sphere, V = $4\pi r^3/3$, and thus the ventricular radius (r) = 4 cm. Then: S = (20 mm Hg)(4 cm)/(2) × (1.5 cm) = 26.7 mm Hg.

4.15. c. All the considerations in the previous question hold here, except that the maximum afterload is requested. Thus, again,

$S = (P_{TM} \times r)/2h$, and as h is defined to be constant in this problem, we must look for S where $P_{TM} \times r$ is a maximum. (We shall have to subtract the preload from the total load to get the afterload.) The equation should lead us to suspect that the S will be greatest when P and/or r are greatest, and thus to confine our calculations to the ejection phase. When the P is 100 mm Hg, 0.8 of the SV (or 40 ml) has been ejected, leaving a volume of 228 ml at that point. The r can be calculated to be 3.79 cm, leading to a total $S = 126.3$ mm Hg. Subtracting the preload of 26.7 mm Hg gives the maximum afterload of 99.6 mm Hg.

4.16. b. Curve 2 demonstrates an enhancement of cardiac function. All the choices except the stimulation of vagal efferent nerves to the heart can bring that about.

4.17. d. Curve 3 demonstrates a decline in cardiac function, which is a common result of cardiac failure.

5

Control of the Circulation

INTRODUCTION

This chapter provides a quick view of circulatory regulation, stressing the big picture. In some cases controversy may be side-stepped in the interests of a straightforward presentation. There is simply no room to present all the pros and cons of this still-evolving field in our introductory text.

Physiologic control of the circulation provides an adequate blood supply to each of an animal's vital organs. This is achieved by three groups of control systems:

1. **systemic** mechanisms keep **mean arterial blood pressure** nearly constant;
2. **local** mechanisms make use of this constant arterial pressure to regulate **individual organ flows;** and
3. **systemic blood volume** is assured by a number of other, more slowly acting systems.

A simplified overall picture of circulatory control is presented in Fig. 5.1. This chapter should help you to understand each of the relationships pictured there.

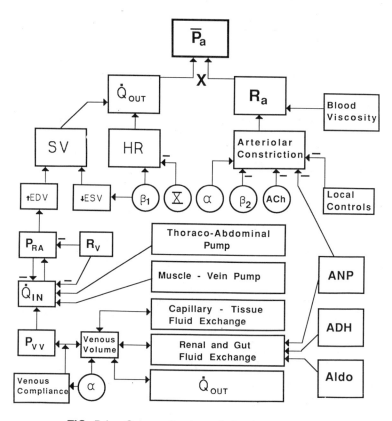

FIG. 5.1. Schematic view of circulatory control.

LOCAL CONTROL MECHANISMS (FOR INDIVIDUAL ORGAN FLOWS)

This discussion of circulatory control will begin with the selfserving local mechanisms that provide a flow appropriate to each organ's needs. These controls work fast, usually within seconds, and can be thought of as vasodilating mechanisms at the arteriolar and precapillary sphincter levels. The general principle tying these mechanisms together is the following: Vasodilation is directly stimulated by the very things that would happen if the circulation were greatly slowed down. That is, vasodilation is promoted:

1. by the accumulation of cellular metabolic products,
2. by a fall in local P_{O_2}, and
3. by the release of intracellular contents from inadequately perfused cells.

The increase in flow that follows vasodilation corrects this situation by washing away the unnatural extracellular inhabitants and bringing more oxygen to the tissue.

Thus, the release of the normally intracellular ions K^+, Mg^{2+}, and HPO_4^- induces vasodilation. Ca^{2+}, on the other hand, is perhaps 5,000-fold higher in concentration outside cells than within, and an increase in its local concentration will promote vasoconstriction instead. Both the CO_2 produced by aerobic metabolism and the lactic acid produced by anaerobic metabolism are important vasodilators. Brain blood flow, for example, is thought to be regulated principally by P_{CO_2} levels. In the heart, and probably in skeletal muscle as well, the release of adenosine following the breakdown of adenosine triphosphate and adenosine diphosphate provokes a physiologically important vasodilation. The coronary circulation vasodilates if local O_2 tensions fall. A local rise in temperature consequent to increased metabolism will lower arteriolar resistance in most tissues.

Strong effects are achieved by locally released histamine, 5-hydroxytryptamine, and bradykinin, all of which tend to **lower** arteriolar resistance, **raise** postcapillary resistance, and increase capillary permeability. These three actions all tend to promote fluid transudation out of the vascular system into tissue extracellular space. The exact physiological role of these agents is not known, however. The prostaglandins and related compounds are currently achieving publicity for their strong vasoactive properties: Those of the E series tend to relax vessels and those of the F series tend to contract vessels. But again, their physiological importance is not well understood. All these agents can act in at least two important ways:

1. directly on arteriolar smooth muscle cells to relax them; and
2. indirectly on these cells by interfering with the local release of the vasoconstrictor, norepinephrine. This hormone is normally

released by sympathetic nervous endings in the vicinity of vascular smooth muscle to maintain vascular tone.

In certain tissues, for example kidney and skeletal muscle, the above mechanisms probably contribute to a phenomenon called autoregulation. This term is used to describe the fact that flow through these tissues remains remarkably constant while perfusing arterial pressures vary from as low as 40 mm Hg to as high as 160 mm Hg.

SYSTEMIC CONTROL MECHANISMS (FOR MEAN ARTERIAL PRESSURE)

Introduction

Millions of dollars have been spent to further our understanding of just how the body controls mean arterial pressure. With such a budget you can bet the answers won't be simple and that they'll get more complicated with each passing year.

Exercise, the consumption of meals, changes in body position, nose bleeds, fever, and other shocks to the body will all act to change our arterial blood pressure unless we do something about it. Yet arterial blood pressure normally varies little from a mean value of 95 mm Hg. Include in this system an independent pump, such that what goes in one end comes out the other **in spite of** arterial pressure (Frank–Starling law of the heart), and one begins to wonder just how the body controls it all.

The body does its job using complex sets of receptors, controllers, and effectors. We'll discuss them as eight different mechanisms, keeping in mind that they interact strongly with one another. A list of the mechanisms is given in Table 5.1. The systems have been arranged from the most rapidly acting ones to those that make adjustments over days. The former defend our blood pressure on a moment-to-moment basis, the latter achieve longer range pressure stability by managing circulating volume. Let's look at them one by one.

TABLE 5.1. *Circulatory Control Mechanisms*

System
Arterial baroreceptors
Peripheral chemoreceptors
Central nervous system ischemic response
Renin–angiotensin
Capillary fluid shifts
Atrial natriuretic peptide
Aldosterone
Antidiuretic hormone

Arterial Baroreceptors

Stretch receptors, located within the walls of the internal carotids and the aortic arch, offer the first line of defense against raised or lowered arterial pressure (Fig. 5.2). When stretched by high transmural pressure these receptors send signals via branches of the glossopharyngeal (carotid impulses) and vagal (aortic impulses) cranial nerves to the central nervous system for processing. The carotid sinus receptors normally begin firing at arterial pressures above about 65–70 mm Hg, and their maximal discharge frequencies are reached by 180 mm Hg. They are sensitive not only to instantaneous pressure levels, but also to the rate of change of pressure, hence rapid pressure wave upswings will produce a higher response at a given mean pressure level. In man the aortic system seems to have a somewhat higher threshold, not firing until pressures of 80–90 mm Hg are reached.

Nevertheless, whereas these receptors and the control system to which they're attached can readjust pressures within a few heartbeats, they also fatigue easily. So, if some nefarious force were to keep mean arterial pressure elevated for a period of several hours, we would find our receptors avidly defending the **new** higher level. In effect, they are easily resettable. When these receptors are absent, an animal's mean blood pressure during a day may be normal, but the swings will be much greater than normal—to both dangerously high and dangerously low levels.

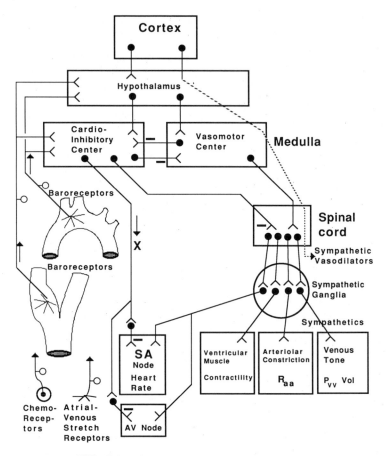

FIG. 5.2.   Autonomic control of circulation.

How do these afferent baroreceptor signals to the central nervous system regulate pressure? First they enter an effective controlling system in the brainstem where they synapse with cells within the nucleus of the solitary tract. There are relays from here to the dorsal vagal nucleus, to the ambiguous nucleus, and to the paramedian reticular nuclei in an incompletely defined area termed the vasomotor center. There is also sensory input to this general area from such diverse sources as pain fibers, the cerebellum, and the cerebral cortex (via the hypothalamus).

Three distinct sorts of motor signals arise in this area in response to "pressure-is-high" baroceptor information:

1. The efferent vagus will **increase** its inhibitory **parasympathetic** signals to the sinus node and conducting system of the heart and act to slow heart rate.

2. The **sympathetic** nervous system will **decrease** normal tonic activity being sent from the vasomotor center to peripheral effectors. At some synapses still within the spinal cord neurons carrying these sympathetic signals release the neurotransmitter norepinephrine. At more peripheral synapses neurons within the paravertebral sympathetic ganglia release the neurotransmitter acetylcholine. Still more peripherally at effector end organs neurons again release norepinephrine. To repeat, this sympathetic output is partly suppressed by baroreceptor signals, which indicate high pressure.

3. A parallel **inhibitory** sympathetic pathway within the spinal cord is also activated. It is thought to **inhibit** what are usually considered to be sympathetic effects. At its last synapses within the spinal cord, this subsystem releases 5-hydroxytryptamine (serotonin) instead of norepinephrine. The norepinephrine released at sympathetic terminals has four important circulatory actions:

1. at the heart's sinus node it increases **heart rate;**
2. within the ventricular mass it increases **heart contractility;**
3. at arterioles in most organs it contracts vascular smooth muscle, increasing **arteriolar resistance;** and
4. at the venular and venous levels it contracts vascular smooth muscle, increasing **venous tone,** thus decreasing venous capacity and delivering more blood to the heart.

All these actions normally tend to promote a higher arterial blood pressure, therefore their suppression by increased baroreceptor signals will tend to lower blood pressure. Effects 1, 2, and 4 above all tend to promote a higher cardiac output ($\dot{Q}$), and 3 increases systemic resistance (R).

Sympathetic nervous outflow also releases acetylcholine in those extra-large sympathetic ganglia commonly known as the adrenal medullae. This in turn stimulates a release of the hormones epinephrine and norepinephrine (in a 4-to-1 ratio), which rapidly find their way into the bloodstream. These adrenal-released hormones seem to be relatively unimportant in overall circulatory management under most physiological circumstances, however.

Peripheral Chemoreceptors

Primarily of importance in the regulation of respiration, the carotid and aortic body chemoreceptors have some influence on the cardiovascular system as well. They are stimulated to fire by low P_{O_2} and to a lesser extent by high P_{CO_2} and low pH. A low perfusing pressure excites all these mechanisms by causing a lower blood flow through the substrate-hungry receptors. In addition, concomitant increases in sympathetic output to the body in general act to increase arteriolar resistance within the chemoreceptors as well, thus further compromising their blood supply. The net result is that local chemoreceptor P_{O_2} is lower and metabolic products accumulate. Low pressure thus produces a higher signal rate to the central nervous system, again via the glossopharyngeal and vagal nerves. In terms of nerve traffic this is the reverse of the baroreceptor situation in which **higher** pressures produce more afferent impulses. Fortunately, the medullary centers sort all this out. The chemoreceptor pressure mechanism does not kick in until mean pressures go below 80 mm Hg, however, so this is a backup system even though it acts quite rapidly. Systemic circulatory effects of this stimulation are those of increased sympathetic outflow and vagal outflow. The net result is systemic vasoconstriction and a tendency toward a **slower** heart rate.

Central Nervous System Ischemic Response

Some cells within the brainstem and perhaps elsewhere in the central nervous system are stimulated to fire by P_{O_2}s lower than 50 mm Hg or so. This can happen not only as a result of low arterial oxygenation but also as a result of low arterial pressures and consequent low cerebrovascular blood flows. The sympathetic output is half-maximal within a half minute or so, and under certain conditions can achieve peripheral levels of sympathetic activity up to seven times that due to the maximal baroreceptor response. This is often only an agonal response, though, because Po_2 levels much lower than this will not usually sustain neuronal activity.

The Renin–Angiotensin System

Renin is released from juxtaglomerular distal tubular cells in the kidney in response to three stimuli:

1. decreased afferent arteriolar pressure,
2. decreased delivery of Na^+ and Cl^- to the distal tubules, and
3. increased efferent discharge of the renal sympathetics.

Renin then acts on its alpha$_2$-globulin substrate to produce the peptide angiotensin I, which is in turn clipped to a shorter peptide, angiotensin II, by an enzyme resident in the endothelial cells of lung capillaries. Besides being an extremely potent vasoconstrictor in its own right, angiotensin II probably produces most of its physiological effects via its potentiation of norepinephrine. Not only does it increase both norepinephrine synthesis in and release from sympathetic endings, it also enhances norepinephrine binding to effector organ cell membrane sites and inhibits its normally rapid reuptake into nerves. It also stimulates thirst centers in the hypothalamus and releases aldosterone (see below) from the adrenal cortex. The release of the powerful vasoconstrictor angiotensin II by the renin system will be discussed in more detail in a renal physiology text. Lower pressures, acting through the release of renin, excite the same mechanisms as the baroreceptor system does. In addition, renin contributes over a longer time scale to blood volume expansion, which in turn acts to increase cardiac input, cardiac output, and hence blood pressure.

Capillary Fluid Shifts

In many physiologic states, such as dehydration and hemorrhage, decreases in arterial pressure are accompanied by decreases in tissue capillary pressure as well. As is discussed on pages 88–90, one of the major forces determining water flow across the capillary endothelium is the transmural hydrostatic pressure gradient. Thus, if capillary pressure is lowered there will be a net influx of water from the tissues into the bloodstream, in effect, a fluid transfusion. The resulting higher vascular volume will act to sustain blood pressure via its enhancement of venous return. The reverse is also true: higher capillary pressures will be buffered by an efflux of water into the tissues.

Atrial Natriuretic Peptide

Very recently, physiologists have discovered another naturally occurring hormone with important circulatory effects in experimental animals. They found at first that injection of extracts from minced atria into the circulation produced a significant loss of salt and water through the kidneys. Further work identified the active principles as small peptides, resident in granules within the atrial tissue. These atrial natriuretic peptides (ANP) appear to be released into the circulation when the atria are stretched, and thus mediate an appropriate response to this volume-overloaded situation by getting rid of excess body fluids. Current investigations are demonstrating additional vasodilating and anti-ADH (ADH = antidiuretic hormone) activity properties of these interesting agents. The jury is still out on the physiological relevance of ANP to circulatory control in humans, but the outlook is promising.

Aldosterone

Maintaining pressure means maintaining extracellular volume as well, and this depends to a large extent on the body's store of

NaCl, the principal extracellular salt. The protagonist in this drama is aldosterone, and its actions are discussed in greater detail in renal physiology texts. Here it is necessary to say only that aldosterone acts at the distal renal tubules to retain Na^+. It is secreted by the adrenal cortex in response to circulating angiotensin II.

Antidiuretic Hormone

Antidiuretic hormone (ADH), also known as vasopressin, is manufactured in the hypothalamus for delivery to the bloodstream from the posterior pituitary. Although it is an extremely potent vasoconstrictor, its main physiologic importance probably derives from its ability to enable the kidney to retrieve water from the renal collecting tubules. Restricting water loss keeps circulating fluid volumes up and is therefore very important in the long-term management of blood pressure.

A major **inhibition** of ADH release occurs when vagal receptor fibers at the junctions of the large veins with the atria are stretched. These volume receptors sense overfilling of the venous compartment of the circulation and by lowering ADH levels allow the excretion of more water. Conversely, when these myelinated afferent vagal fibers are **less** stretched than normal the decreased receptor firing will promote the retention of water.

In addition, these same vagal afferents produce a mixed bag of autonomic effects via the vasomotor center. Whereas sympathetic impulses to the sinoatrial (SA) node are **increased,** thereby increasing heart rate, other sympathetic impulses to renal afferent arterioles and to systemic arterioles in general are **decreased.** These actions are appropriate in that volume overloading of the atria would be relieved by higher heart rates, and circulatory volume itself would be lowered by movement of water across capillaries into tissues and out into the urine.

There are some unmyelinated atrial vagal fibers that act like typical arterial baroreceptors when stretched. In some ways their actions may be contrary to those of their myelinated cousins.

SUMMARY

Circulatory pressure and volume are the most important dependent variables in regulation of the circulation. Pressure is defended acutely (within seconds to minutes), whereas volume adjustments are made on a slower time scale (within minutes to days). Both pressure and volume interact with each other directly via vascular compliances and indirectly through volume and pressure receptors, so they are not controlled in isolation. Once each organ is guaranteed a reasonable arterial perfusing pressure it can select its own appropriate flow by altering local arteriolar resistance.

QUESTIONS

5.01. Sudden inflation of sphygmomanometer cuffs about both thighs to a pressure of 300 mm Hg in a normal, resting, recumbent person would be expected, when a new steady state has been achieved, to have produced the greatest rise in:

a. Right atrial pressure.
b. Total peripheral resistance.
c. Cardiac output.
d. Aortic pressure.
e. Pulmonary blood flow.

5.02. Decreasing pressure around the outside of one carotid sinus would:

a. Have the same effect as cutting the carotid sinus nerve.
b. Reflexly slow heart rate and cause peripheral vasodilation.
c. Speed both heart rate and respiratory frequency.
d. Increase blood flow to the brain.
e. Increase the slope of the prepotential in the sinoatrial node.

5.03. The rate of firing of carotid baroreceptors is likely to be increased as a result of:

a. A prolonged forced expiratory effort against a closed glottis.
b. Hemorrhage.
c. An increase in pulse pressure.
d. A decrease in peripheral resistance.
e. Dehydration.

5.04. A fall in systemic arterial pressure produced, for example, by suddenly getting out of a hot tub and standing motionless, is most likely to result in a reflexly induced:

a. Slowing of the heart rate and arteriolar dilation.
b. Slowing of the heart rate and arteriolar constriction.
c. Speeding of the heart rate and arteriolar dilation.
d. Speeding of the heart rate and arteriolar constriction.
e. Decrease in venous tone.

Figure 5.3 shows a lead II EKG. At the arrow, some physiological or pharmacological change was instituted. The time scale is as shown at the top. Use the record to answer **Questions 5.05–5.07.**

5.05. The record after the arrow shows:

a. First-degree atrioventricular block.
b. Second-degree atrioventricular block.
c. Third-degree atrioventricular block.
d. Atrial fibrillation.
e. Sinus tachycardia.

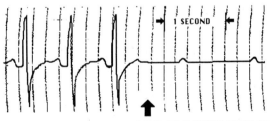

LEAD II EKG. AT THE ARROW, SOME PHYSIOLOGICAL OR PHARMACOLOGICAL CHANGE WAS INSTITUTED. TIME SCALE IS AS SHOWN AT THE TOP OF THE RECORD.

FIG. 5.3. See Questions 5.05–5.07.

5.06. You can confidently conclude that, after the arrow:

a. The P_{MC} was falling.
b. The right atrial pressure was rising.
c. First heart sounds continued to occur.
d. Second heart sounds continued to occur.
e. The arterial pulse could still be felt, although at a slower rate.

5.07. All of the following might have caused the change at the arrow EXCEPT:

a. Stimulation of the right vagus nerve.
b. Stimulation of the left vagus nerve.
c. Sudden increase of the pressure within a carotid sinus.
d. Sudden increase of pressure around (outside of) one carotid sinus.
e. Sudden decrease of pressure around (outside of) one carotid sinus.

Answer Questions **5.08–5.10** by selecting the EXPERIMENTAL MANIPULATION (A–E below) that would produce the indicated result.

A. Section of the vagus and carotid sinus nerves.
B. Inhalation of 5% CO_2.
C. Stimulation of sympathetic nerves to the heart.
D. Injection of norepinephrine.
E. Stimulation of carotid sinus nerves.

5.08. ___ would decrease cerebral vascular resistance.

5.09. ___ would lower mean arterial pressure and heart rate.

5.10. ___ would elevate mean arterial pressure and impair postural circulatory reflexes.

ANSWERS

5.01. b. The cuffs will prevent inflow to—or outflow from— the legs, and, the blood volume associated with the legs' vessels would be sequestered there. Insofar as the cardiovascular system is concerned, the legs would have been amputated. There is no reason to believe that either the aortic pressure or the right atrial pressure would change. The cardiac output and the pulmonary blood flow must be equal to one another, and must be reduced in proportion to the part of the circulation which has been "amputated." Only the total peripheral resistance would increase. If the resistance of the leg vessels had been $\frac{1}{3}$ of the total in the control situation, the total resistance in the cuffed situation must be $\frac{3}{2}$ what it was before.

5.02. b. The carotid sinus transmural pressure ($P_{TM} = P_{in} - P_{out}$) is the pressure which distends it. Thus, decreasing the P outside the vessel will distend it more, and will have the same effect on the baroreceptors as will an increase in arterial pressure.

5.03. c. Choices a, b, d, and e will all tend to reduce arterial pressure. $P_{Ao} - P_{RA} = R \times \dot{Q}$. Choice d will reduce the R term directly, and choices a, b, and e will all reduce venous return and thus $\dot{Q}$. The baroreceptors are sensitive to the arterial pulse pressure as well as the mean arterial pressure.

5.04. d. The baroreceptors will tend to resist the decrease in arterial pressure.

5.05. c. There are P waves but there are no QRSs.

5.06. b. When ventricular activity ceases, all cardiovascular system pressures begin to approach the P_{MC}. Thus, arterial pressures will fall and P_{RA} will rise.

5.07. d. Choices a and b would cause the changes directly. Choices c and e can do so via the carotid sinus reflex. Choice d will, if anything, cause the opposite changes.

5.08. B. The brain circulation is strongly vasodilated by elevated P_{CO_2}.

5.09. E. Stimulating carotid sinus nerves sends the same sort of message to the brain as does raising the arterial pressure.

5.10. A. Cutting the vagus nerves denervates the aortic baroreceptors and prevents parasympathetic efferent nerves from influencing the heart. Cutting the carotid sinus nerves denervates the carotid sinus baroreceptors. The sudden removal of any impulse traffic in the baroreceptor afferents is the same message the brain would get if the arterial pressure were to fall drastically. It thus leads to a dramatic increase in the arterial pressure. The postural circulatory reflexes are impaired because the baroreceptor reflexes are essential in opposing the changes in arterial pressure caused by changes in position.

6

Circulation through Individual Organs

INTRODUCTION

In contrast to the last section which dealt with circulatory control mechanisms in general, this section focuses on the peculiarities of blood circulation through individual organs. Each organ's circulation is adjusted to its special needs, while allowing circulation to the heart and brain first priority as necessary. In the subsections below, we'll discuss some of the special circulatory problems facing the body's major organs.

Skin Circulation

The skin, a 2-kg organ, keeps foreign materials from penetrating the body, stops precious body fluids from escaping too fast, and allows the regulated dissipation of heat produced by our metabolism. This last function is achieved in the outer 1 mm of the skin by a well-designed radiator system consisting of an extensive network of venules. When blood is allowed into these superficial venules it readily loses its heat to the outside (if the outside temperature is colder than it is). If blood is not allowed to flow into the region this outer portion of the skin acts as an efficient insulator, preventing excess heat loss. The result is usually preservation of the core body temperature at which the brain, heart, and other organs can function optimally.

There are two effectors allowing blood to flow into the venular plexus:

1. Skin arterioles and
2. arteriovenous (a-v) shunts.

The latter are structures 20–40 μm in diameter, by-passing normal capillary beds. They are found principally in our five extremities: the feet, the hands, and the head.

How does the body regulate blood flow into this venular radiator? There are two known temperature sensing receptors in our system:

1. one set centrally located in the anterior hypothalamus, and
2. another set within the skin itself.

The former measures core temperatures, the latter anticipates problems by sensing environmental temperatures. The core receptors have perhaps 10 times as much gain (produce 10 times the effect per degree temperature rise) as the peripheral sensors. Both receptor sets are hooked up to medullary cardiovascular centers which control sympathetic outflow to the a-v shunts and arterioles. Alpha receptors in these effector structures respond to the local release of norepinephrine.

In addition to the above neurally connected system, local temperature rises will also serve to dilate arterioles and a-v shunts. At 40°C and above this local mechanism will uncouple the central neural control, and thereby take over completely. There is also evidence for an active neural vasodilator mechanism operating on skin arterioles. The whole system is dependent upon arterial blood pressure for its function as well. With all these potential control mechanisms competing, temperature regulation can be a complex process.

What sorts of changes can the system produce? At rest in a thermally neutral environment about 0.5 L/min (9%) of our cardiac output flows through the skin. This can be decreased to as low as 20 ml/min or increased to as high as 8 L/min, a 400-fold variation overall, with an even greater relative range in our extremities.

The corresponding variation in heat flux across the skin is from 0.02 to 30 kCal/min.

A more complete discussion of temperature regulation is beyond the scope of this circulatory section, but perhaps you can now see the central role played by this peripheral organ in maintaining body homeostasis.

SKELETAL MUSCLE CIRCULATION

Skeletal muscle's main job is to perform work on the environment. It is not perfused as generously at rest as during exercise.

Resting skeletal muscle consumes only 20% of the total body $\dot{V}O_2$ (50 out of 250 ml O_2/min) even though it constitutes roughly 45% (30 out of 70 kg) of our total body mass. Just how much blood flow ($\dot{Q}$) is supplied to resting skeletal muscle, and therefore just how much O_2 is extracted at rest from each liter of that $\dot{Q}$ is a matter of some controversy at present. Some investigators report a $\dot{Q}$ of 1.1 L/min in association with an arteriovenous difference of 45 ml O_2/L blood. The venous blood O_2 content of 155 ml O_2/L blood would correspond to a venous PO_2 of more than 40 mm Hg. Others contend that these measurements were made in the presence of sympathetic vasodilation of skeletal muscle, which is hard to avoid, and that the measurements may therefore not be valid. These latter workers report a $\dot{Q}$ of only 0.5 L/min in resting skeletal muscle, resulting in an O_2 extraction of about 100 ml O_2/L blood, a venous O_2 content of about 100 ml O_2/L blood, and a venous PO_2 of about 25–30 mm Hg. The issue is not yet resolved.

In maximal exercise, muscle $\dot{V}O_2$ can be as much as 60-fold higher than at rest, with changes taking place almost immediately upon demand. Even this greatly increased O_2 delivery won't produce enough energy in many cases, and the muscle will generate some adenosine triphosphate anerobically, repaying its oxygen debt later during a rest period. To supply this vastly increased O_2 flux, two basic mechanisms are available:

1. an **increased extraction** of O_2 from the blood so that muscle venous blood now will be quite "blue" at a content as low as 40 ml O_2/L blood (80% extraction), and
2. an **increased flow** of O_2-carrying blood.

The **increased extraction** occurs because of changing Po_2 gradients. The **increased blood flow** is the mechanism concerning us here. How is it achieved?

First of all, arterioles in muscles at rest have a high basal tone, explaining a major portion of resting vascular resistance. This tone can be transiently overcome by active sympathetic vasodilation, but this mechanism usually comes into play as an **anticipation** of exercise, and lasts less than a minute. The principle **vasodilating agents,** however, seem to the the local metabolites released by increased muscle activity. Thus H^+, CO_2, K^+, Mg^{2+}, and adenosine are all powerful vasodilators and act to increase muscle blood flow during exercise.

Bear in mind that heavy muscle exercise is usually accompanied by substantially increased **sympathetic nervous activity** and that a general effect of this is to stimulate alpha receptors everywhere in the body. In active muscle this would be counterproductive, tending to reduce the blood supply. This doesn't happen, however, because the alpha effect is wiped out by the competing local vasodilating mechanisms. Elsewhere, alpha receptor stimulation lowers blood flows, effectively shunting blood from inactive tissue to active muscles.

Also playing a role in delivering O_2 to active muscle cells is the rapid opening of capillary networks, termed **capillary recruitment.** This enhances O_2 delivery principally through the much shorter O_2 diffusion paths that result.

Active and **sustained muscle contraction,** as in weightlifting for example, tend to impede muscle blood flow transiently, giving rise to higher systemic resistances and therefore higher blood pressures. The rhythmic exercise of bicycling or running, on the other hand, will not raise blood pressure significantly.

CORONARY CIRCULATION

The heart is always an actively exercising muscle. Even at rest its oxygen extraction is very large, producing some of the bluest blood the body knows. As the coronary blood flow at rest is about 0.25 L/min and its $\dot{V}O_2$ is about 27 ml O_2/min, the Fick principle allows us to calculate an arteriovenous O_2 concentration difference of about 110 ml O_2/L blood ($CaO_2 - CvO_2 = \dot{V}O_2/\dot{Q} = $ (27 ml O_2/min)/(0.25 L blood/min) = 110 ml O_2/L blood). This means the coronary circulation is extracting 55% (100 × 110/200) of the O_2 passing through it, practically a maximal value that isn't increased under normal circumstances. To get more O_2 the heart normally has to increase the flow of blood delivering that O_2. Another problem common to heart muscle and exercising skeletal muscle has to do with compression of the circulation during contraction. In the heart this happens once every heart beat (during systole), and it means that coronary perfusion is effectively limited to diastole.

Let's consider these two problems in a bit more detail before going on to discuss how the heart manages to increase coronary flow as the demand for $\dot{V}O_2$ increases. First of all, **cardiac O_2 extraction** is near maximal at rest and therefore can't improve much during periods of increased O_2 demand. As noted above in the discussion of skeletal muscle, the only physiological way to increase local $\dot{V}O_2$ is to increase the blood flow through the tissue, so this mechanism becomes of critical importance to heart muscle. Impeding the flow with atherosclerotic arterial plaques is likely to cause problems.

Systole provides a natural impediment to forward blood flow. Within the actively contracting endocardial muscle, where perivascular pressures are highest during contraction, there is a negative (or at most zero) gradient of pressure across the walls of blood vessels. This pressure gradient tends to squeeze the vessels shut when the heart itself is squeezing. It is not unusual to be able to record an actual reversal of flow in the large epicardial coronary arteries as blood is pushed backward (see Fig. 6.1). This is particu-

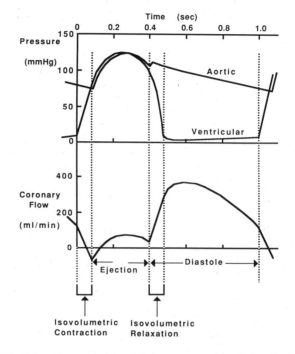

FIG. 6.1. Coronary blood flow occurs primarily in diastole.

larly evident during systolic isometric contraction, when aortic pressure, tending to push blood forward, is at its lowest, and muscle wall stress, tending to squeeze the muscle, is near its highest. The problem is greatest for the deepest, most endocardial muscle adjacent to the high-pressure left ventricular chamber.

What about the His–Purkinje conduction system and the papillary muscle connections to the wall? Both of these lie practically within the chamber. Shouldn't chamber pressure keep them from receiving O_2 and functioning properly? There is evidence that these structures can exchange O_2 and other diffusable materials directly with ventricular blood. The innermost 1 mm or so of the myocardium is in this way supplemented by supplies that don't have to traverse the coronaries. Purkinje system conduction defects are common in cases of coronary arterial occlusion, though, so this system isn't a perfect substitute.

The message should be clear: Cumulative diastolic time is necessary for cumulative coronary flow, and nothing else will do to supply O_2. Remember that exercise increases heart rates by shortening diastolic time more than systolic time, so this factor limits our cardiac function during maximal exercise. Not surprisingly, high heart rates are poorly tolerated by patients with coronary artery disease.

How does the coronary circulation cope with an increased demand for O_2 as diastolic time is shortened? Because different regions of the heart will simultaneously have different needs, the solution has been a kind of "local option." Overall autonomic nervous influences are far less important than the highly localized release of vasodilator substances and the localized production of low P_{O_2}. Of these mechanisms, adenosine release and low P_{O_2} seem to be the most important for vasodilation, but this is an expanding area of research so the story may change.

The vasodilation of arterioles isn't the whole picture. Recruitment of closed capillary channels is equally important, lowering O_2 gradients by decreasing the length of O_2 diffusion paths. Cells at the end of the diffusion line won't be robbed by hungry cells along the way if the lines are kept short. In those people fortunate enough to be born with good right-to-left coronary arterial anastamoses or in those lucky enough to be given time to develop them, the partial occlusion of a large branch of the left coronary artery will be partly compensated by flow via the right coronary artery.

The big picture of the coronary circulation is therefore one of local autonomy. This doesn't mean that systemic hormones and drugs and nervous influences can't be important in extreme cases. When insufficient O_2 is being delivered to a heart it will perish unless we find ways to decrease the demand for O_2 or to remove any pathological circulatory block. Chances are in most pathological states the coronary circulation is already doing all it can and vasodilator therapy would be ineffectual.

CEREBRAL CIRCULATION

What systemic circulatory controls does the brain need? Give it adequate arterial pressure and enough blood nearly saturated with O_2 and it can be left to itself. This organ needs protection above all others, so there is no reason to constrict its arterioles when systemic blood pressure falls.

On the other hand, brain function requires very large changes in local flow depending upon which part of the brain is working, so reasonably **sensitive local vasodilator mechanisms** are called for. Vasodilation, and hence increased brain blood flow, follows an increase in Pco_2 or a decrease in O_2, which probably act via decreased extracellular pH. Other local neural vasodilator mechanisms may also play a role, although the evidence is less certain.

Probably related to these local vasodilator responses is the observation that brain blood flow shows good **autoregulation,** that is, overall brain blood flow changes remarkably little as mean arterial pressure varies from about 75 mm Hg to 180 mm Hg.

It is thought that **capillary recruitment** also plays a significant role in supplying O_2 to brain cells because brains are extremely rich in these vessels. These brain capillaries are different from many in the body in that they have no slit pores. This and their rich neuroglial investment make them poorly permeable to salts and virtually impermeable to proteins: a blood–brain barrier. One functional significance of this barrier is that excess water can more easily be kept out of the extravascular space. Trapped inside a rigid skull, such fluid can (and does on occasion) compress vessels and lead to substantially decreased cerebral blood flow. When this occurs, stretch receptors in certain cerebral arteries act like baroreceptors and reflexly cause systemic blood pressure to rise, opposing the compression.

Cerebral blood flow averages 750 ml/min in adults, and brain $\dot{V}o_2$ is 48 ml O_2/min, yielding an a-v difference of 64 ml O_2/L. Cortical gray matter uses even more blood and O_2 per weight and time than the working heart, which may be why brain cells don't have the recovery potential of cells from skin, muscle, or kidney. Even brief (10 min) interruptions in blood supply can have disastrous consequences. Vasospasm due to calcium leakage into cells may play a role in this response to cerebral circulatory arrest, and calcium-blocking drugs have been able to ameliorate its effects considerably.

SPLANCHNIC CIRCULATION

The circulation to the gastrointestinal (GI) tract, spleen, and liver is tuned to the function of these organs, but is **subject to interruption** when blood volume and flow are needed elsewhere. For example, the sympathetic outflow associated with maximal exercise can take effectively 80% of the resting gut blood flow and divert it to more pressing needs. The splanchnic organs temporarily make do with less blood flow and finish their jobs later.

At rest in the supine position the GI tract and associated structures take a fair share of the cardiac output (1.4 L/min, 25%) and total $\dot{V}O_2$ (56 ml O_2/min, 27%). Merely assuming the upright position lowers these figures as some blood pooling in the extremities is countered by a diversion of splanchnic flow. The arteriovenous O_2 difference calculated from these figures (40 ml O_2/L blood) indicates that these tissues don't normally remove a large share of the O_2 from the blood, and that they have a fair reserve to draw upon, much like skeletal muscle.

Both the volume (25% of total) and flow of blood can be diverted to maintain perfusion of the brain and heart when pressure falls and to maintain perfusion of skeletal muscle and skin during exercise.

When not being stimulated by central sympathetics the gut is able to increase its mucosal blood flow eightfold during the water secretion phase of digestion. Such an increase is necessary to prevent excess local hemoconcentration and greatly increased viscosity as water is lost from the blood. When large water or solute fluxes across the gut mucosa are not necessary, solute/water activity gradients between circulating blood and gut lumen are maintained by slow flow in the **countercurrent circulation** consisting of central arterioles and returning capillary network present in the villi of the gut mucosa. When blood flow is increased the countercurrent mechanism is washed out, and the large surface area of the villi becomes available for secretion or absorption. At the same time the increased blood flow delivers or carries away the solutes or water involved.

Blood leaving the gut enters the liver via the portal vein at a pressure of 8–12 mm Hg. Here the flow is augmented in humans by a small contribution from the hepatic artery.

RENAL CIRCULATION

The kidneys' job is to remove waste products from the blood and excrete them. To do this they have to filter some 120 ml of plasma water-plus-solutes each minute without unduly concentrating the remaining red cells and protein. To do this, approximately 25% of the cardiac output at rest is sent through the kidneys, although these organs make up only 0.5% of our mass. The flow is in excess of metabolic needs, inasmuch as the arteriovenous O_2 difference is only 15 ml O_2/L blood.

During exercise and at other times of general circulatory need the kidneys are deprived of much of their normal blood flow by afferent arteriolar constriction caused by increased sympathetic activity. In fact, one clue that a patient is in circulatory shock is that no urine is being excreted. Prolonged deprivation of the blood supply in such cases will lead to renal failure.

In the laboratory during periods of artificially controlled, steady sympathetic tone, the kidney shows strong **autoregulation,** that is, flow remains reasonably constant while the mean arterial blood pressure is varied between about 50 and 150 mm Hg. Naturally, in an intact animal, this process would be hard to demonstrate because low pressures would cause afferent renal arteriolar constriction via the baroreceptor reflex. These experiments do demonstrate, however, that even the renal circulation has local mechanisms that try to maintain flow under adverse circumstances.

PULMONARY CIRCULATION

The lung is a complicated organ with complicated tasks to perform. Practically all of the cardiac output circulates through it via the pulmonary artery, and an additional preoxygenated supply enters via the bronchial arteries. A small flow is normally shunted around it through the coronary artery–Thebesian vein circuit, which exits into the left ventricular cavity, and through regions of the lung with low ventilation-to-perfusion ratios. Such shunts produce a normal difference of 5–8 mm Hg between the P_{O_2}s of alveolar air and arterial blood. Blood entering the pulmonary circulation leaves by way of the pulmonary veins: There appears to be no functional bronchial venous flow.

The lung circulation has **special requirements:** Increased flow during exercise, deployment of blood from the intrathoracic reservoir when needed elsewhere, and regional matching of pulmonary perfusion to ventilation seem to be the most important.

The first two of these features are closely linked because an excess flow into the lung quickly causes an excess accumulation of blood in the pulmonary circulation, and a deficient flow causes a deficit there. When one stands up suddenly, that extra amount of blood that fills your legs has just been withdrawn from the pulmonary circulation. **The Frank–Starling effect** serves to balance pulmonary and systemic circulations by linking the output of each ventricle to the fullness of its immediately adjacent venous compartment. So, within a few heartbeats, even exercise-induced increases in systemic flow are matched on the pulmonary side. This situation is aided by the fact that changes in heart contractility tend to occur in both ventricles simultaneously. During exercise, lung capillary recruitment acts both to provide additional parallel flow pathways and to distribute flow to well-ventilated areas.

The $\dot{V}_A/\dot{Q}$, or ventilation/perfusion matching problem, is a serious one, particularly in patients who have impaired ventilation or diseased pulmonary circulations. In upright man, gravitational effects cause the $\dot{V}_A/\dot{Q}$ ratio to vary from 3 in the upper upper lobes to

0.6 in the lower lower lobes. Because most ventilation and perfusion at rest occur in the lower lobes, the average is 0.8. During exercise, as higher levels within the lung are ventilated better, the increase in local blood Po_2 there acts to distribute blood flow **toward** this region by direct vasodilation. This is the opposite of what occurs in skeletal muscle, but then the lung is doing just the opposite with the O_2 it is handling. Bear in mind that any ventilation/perfusion mismatch will show up as an A–a (Alveolar–arterial) Po_2 gradient. Abnormalities of this sort are the commonest cause of A–a gradients in excess of 10 mm Hg.

In all of these circulatory adjustments lung capillary pressure must be kept below approximately 25 mm Hg or some fluid will leave the circulation, forming perivascular cuffs, and then actually enter and fill up alveolar air spaces. **Pulmonary edema,** as this is called, occurs frequently in cases of left ventricular failure, in which a competent right ventricle may literally flood the lung. A common time for the appearance of pulmonary edema is after the patient has been lying supine for an hour or more. Some of the circulating blood volume has been moved from the legs to the chest, where it raises local intravascular pressures. This stiffens the lung and may move fluid into alveoli, producing shortness of breath (termed paroxysmal nocturnal dyspnea). Symptoms are usually relieved when the patient sits or stands up, redistributing the offending fluid back to his legs.

PROBLEMS

6.01. Elevated Pa_{CO_2} tends to do all of the following except:

    a. constrict cerebral arterioles by direct action of CO_2 locally.

    b. constrict pulmonary arterioles by direct action of CO_2 locally.

    c. dilate coronary arterioles by direct action of CO_2 locally.

    d. reflexly stimulate sympathetic vasoconstrictor fibers.

    e. raise the systemic arterial pressure.

6.02. Hyperventilation can make one dizzy primarily because it brings about:

a. Increased venous return and thus increased cardiac output.
b. Respiratory acidosis causing increased cerebral blood flow.
c. Hypocapnia causing decreased cerebral blood flow.
d. An elevated O_2 content in arterial blood.
e. A drying out of the respiratory passages.

6.03. In a normal heart, left ventricular coronary blood flow is:

a. less than right ventricular coronary blood flow.
b. reduced during diastole.
c. primarily controlled by sympathetic innervation of coronary arterioles.
d. increased following a fall in Po_2 in the myocardium.
e. greatest during the peak of ventricular systole.

Use Fig. 6.2, representing blood flow into a left coronary artery under normal physiological circumstances, to answer **Questions 6.04–6.07.**

6.04. The period of reverse flow is probably coincident with a period of:

a. rapid ventricular filling.
b. systolic ejection.
c. prolonged coughing.
d. isovolumetric contraction.
e. isovolumetric relaxation.

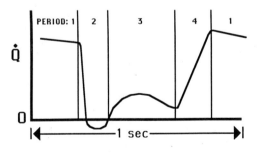

FIG. 6.2. See Questions 6.04–6.07.

6.05. The period of most rapidly increasing flow is probably coincident with a period of:

a. rapid ventricular filling.   d. isovolumetric contraction.
b. systolic ejection.   e. isovolumetric relaxation.
c. prolonged coughing.

6.06. The mitral valve closes:

a. at the line between periods 1 and 2.
b. at the line between periods 2 and 3.
c. at the line between periods 3 and 4.
d. at the line between periods 4 and 1.
e. not at any line but in period 1.

6.07. The aortic valve closes:

a. at the line between periods 1 and 2.
b. at the line between periods 2 and 3.
c. at the line between periods 3 and 4.
d. at the line between periods 4 and 1.
e. not at any line but in period 3.

6.08. At skin temperatures below 40°C, skin blood flow is influenced strongly by the:

a. metabolic rate of the skin.   d. temperature of the hypothalamus.
b. P_{O_2} of the skin.   e. temperature of the basal ganglia.
c. P_{CO_2} of the skin.

6.09. Blood flow in skeletal muscle is increased by all of the following except:

a. decreased tissue P_{O_2} in the muscle.
b. increased tissue P_{CO_2} in the muscle.
c. decreased tissue pH in the muscle.
d. increased extracellular $[K^+]$ in the muscle.
e. norepinephrine acting on alpha adrenergic receptors on arteriolar smooth muscle.

6.10. A normal, resting 70-kg male's cardiac output is 5.5 L/min and his renal oxygen consumption is 20 ml/min. His renal venous (rv) [O_2] in ml O_2/L blood, is closest to:

a. 150
b. 164
c. 182
d. 193
e. 196

6.11. Of the following, the most important determinant of renal blood flow is:

a. renal tissue P_{O_2}.
b. renal tissue P_{CO_2}.
c. the sympathetic nervous system.
d. the amount of glucose delivered to the kidney per minute.
e. the amount of Na^+ delivered to the kidney per minute.

6.12. $\dot{V}_A/\dot{Q}$ mismatching in normal, healthy lungs contributes significantly toward:

a. pulmonary blood flow being greater than systemic blood flow.
b. pulmonary artery pressure being greater than aortic pressure.
c. pulmonary vascular resistance being greater than systemic vascular resistance.
d. alveolar P_{CO_2} being greater than arterial P_{CO_2}.
e. alveolar P_{O_2} being greater than arterial P_{O_2}.

6.13. An increase in $\dot{Q}$ to a given region of the lung can be caused by which of the following changes in that region?

a. increased P_{CO_2}.
b. increased P_{O_2}.
c. elevating the region above the heart.
d. increased airway resistance.
e. decreased lung compliance.

ANSWERS

6.01. a. Elevated Pa_{CO_2} dilates cerebral arterioles.

6.02. c. As above. Hyperventilation decreases alveolar, arterial, and brain P_{CO_2}. The brain vessels are thus caused to constrict, lowering cerebral blood flow. Lowered cerebral blood flow compromises cerebral function, causing dizziness.

6.03. d. A decrease in myocardial P_{O_2} is a very powerful dilater of coronary arterioles.

6.04. d. The critical factors determining coronary blood flow are the driving pressure (Pao $-$ Pv) and the coronary vascular resistance (Rc). Pao is highest during ejection, but Rc is enormous then because the contraction squeezes vessels shut. At the beginning of diastole the Pao is still quite high, and Rc is quite low. During isovolumetric contraction, the Pao is at its lowest, and the contraction squeezes vessels shut, increasing resistance. (See Fig. 6.2).

6.05. e. See answer to 6.04.

6.06. a. Isovolumetric contraction occurs during period 2. The shutting of the mitral valve begins that phase.

6.07. c. Ejection occurs during period 3 and isovolumetric relaxation occurs in period 4. The shutting of the aortic valve separates those two phases.

6.08. d. The temperatures of the hypothalamus and the skin are the two strongest influences on skin blood flow.

6.09. e. Norepinephrine acting on alpha adrenergic receptors constricts vessels.

6.10. c. Use the Fick principle here. Remember that arterial blood normally has about 200 ml O_2/L blood, and that the kidneys

(k) normally receive about 1/5 of the cardiac output. $\dot{Q}_k = \dot{V}_{O_2}/(Ca_{O_2} - Crv_{O_2})$. Then, $Crv_{O_2} = Ca_{O_2} - \dot{V}_{O_2}/\dot{Q}_k = 200$ ml O_2/L blood $-$ (20 ml O_2/min)/(1.1 L blood/min) $= 200$ ml O_2/L blood $- 18$ ml O_2/L blood $= 182$ ml O_2/L blood.

6.11. c. $\dot{Q}_k$ can be decreased or stopped in an attempt to maintain blood pressure.

6.12. e. The two main contributors to a difference between $P_{A_{O_2}}$ and Pa_{O_2} at sea level are the $\dot{V}_A/\dot{Q}$ mismatching and some small amount of right-to-left shunting.

6.13. b. An increased P_{O_2} or a decreased P_{CO_2} acts directly on pulmonary vessels to dilate them, and tends to increase $\dot{Q}$ to that region. Alternatives d and e would lead to decreased $\dot{V}_A$ and thus to increased P_{CO_2} and decreased P_{O_2}.

7

Pathophysiological Exercises

INTRODUCTION

In each case presentation below, the salient symptoms and signs suggesting pathophysiology are denoted by numbers in parentheses like this **(0)**. In other instances, a direct question will be marked by such a number, and in other cases a physiological variable to be calculated will be so indicated. Try to (a) discern the physiological basis of each symptom and sign as it is presented, (b) answer each direct question, and (c) do each indicated calculation, before turning to the Answer section following the case. There you will find corresponding brief explanations and numerical answers. Merely referring to the answers without exercising your intuition and common sense will save you a lot of time, but will keep you from learning to use your newly acquired physiological knowledge.

PATIENT A

Chief Complaint

Mr. A, a 55-year-old electrician, was admitted to University Hospital complaining of tiredness that regularly occurred during his weekly round of golf over the previous 6 months **(1)**.

Present Illness

For 3 years Mr. A had noticed occasional heart palpitations **(2)** which never bothered him. He had no history of shortness of breath, either on exertion **(3)** or at night in bed **(4)**, no chest pain **(5)**, no dizziness **(6)**, and no swelling of his ankles **(7)**.

Past History

There was no family history of heart disease or high blood pressure **(8)**, and he had had no physical exam within the past 20 years **(9)**.

Physical Exam

Mr. A appeared to be a white male of about his stated age in no distress **(10)**. His weight was 75 kg, temp. 37°C, pulse 76/min and regular **(11)**, and blood pressure (left arm, sitting) was 104/67 mm Hg **(12)**. His lungs were clear to auscultation **(13)**, and there was no edema of his extremities **(14)** or hepatospleno-megaly **(15)**. There was a prominent thrust at the cardiac apex **(16)**, but the heart did not appear enlarged **(17)**. There was a grade 3/6 systolic crescendo–decrescendo (so-called ejection) murmur best heard in the second right interspace near the sternum **(18)** with radiation to the neck **(19)**. (Murmurs are usually caused by: (a) a normal flow of blood through a narrowed orifice, for example, pulmonic valve stenosis, (b) an increased flow of blood through a normal orifice, for example, the extra left-to-right shunted blood of an atrial septal defect going out the pulmonic valve, or (c) a high velocity flow of blood going through an unusual orifice, for example, a ventricular septal defect.) The second heart sound was soft **(20)**.

Working Hypothesis

It is usual before ordering laboratory tests to sit back and think about what pathophysiology the patient might have. Consider the possibilities **(21)**.

Laboratory

White cell count and differential and serum LDH (lactic dehydrogenase, released into the circulation by sick or dying muscle cells) were within normal limits **(22)**. Chest X-ray films showed a heart of normal size and contour and clear lung fields **(23)**. The electrocardiogram showed high QRS voltages and slightly depressed ST segments in the left precordial leads **(24)**.

Working Hypothesis

What new pathophysiological information did these laboratory tests contribute **(25)?** What would you expect to find on a two-dimensional echocardiogram, which can show the kinetic anatomy of the heart? Make your prediction before reading the next paragraph.

Echocardiogram

The echocardiogram was consistent with longstanding aortic valvular stenosis: thick left ventricular walls with a thick aortic valve possessing a narrow orifice. It was important at this time that the study ruled out a functional narrowing of the left ventricle (LV) outflow tract by septal hypertrophy in the absence of valvular stenosis. The treatment for such pathology differs greatly from that for valvular stenosis.

Cardiac Catheterization

At this point many physicians would opt for operation without further study of the patient. However, Mr. A was scheduled for cardiac catheterization to confirm the working diagnosis and also to visualize his coronary arterial tree. Before looking at the data presented in Table 7.1, predict what the cardiac catheterization will show. At cardiac catheterization one can measure pressures and oxygen contents in veins, arteries, and the heart chambers. In addition, the use of a radio-opaque dye enables one to outline the coronary arterial tree.

Use the data presented in Table 7.1 to calculate:

Pulmonary blood flow (L/min) **(26)**
Pulmonary vascular resistance [mm Hg/(L/min)] **(27)**
Systemic blood flow (L/min) **(28)**
Cardiac index [(L/min)/m^2] **(29)**
Systemic vascular resistance [mm Hg/(L/min)] **(30)**
Left ventricular stroke volume (ml) **(31)**

Referring to the table of cardiac catheterization data in Table 7.1, are any of the O_2 contents abnormal? How does this help in limiting the diagnostic possibilities **(32)**?

Are any of the pressures abnormal? What do these values contribute to your understanding **(33)**?

What is the possible significance of the calculated systemic flow and cardiac index **(34)**?

What is the significance of the calculated systemic vascular resistance **(35)**?

A pressure tracing from Mr. A's record is shown in Fig. 7.1. From part A of this figure determine the length of time from the peak of the EKG R wave to the peak of the LV pressure wave. Compare this interval with the time between the peak of the R wave and the peak of the aortic pressure tracing in Fig. 7.1B. What do you conclude **(36)**? What do you conclude from a comparison of peak LV and aortic pressures during systole **(37)**?

Calculate a weighted mean pressure for the aorta, assuming that diastolic pressure contributes ⅔ and systolic pressure contributes ⅓. Why does this calculated value differ from the reported mean value of 84 mm Hg **(38)**?

Using the LV pressures and stroke volume obtained at cardiac catheterization, and assuming an LV end-diastolic volume of 105 ml, construct a pressure/volume diagram for the left ventricle **(39)**.

What should be done for this patient **(40)**?

TABLE 7.1. *Cardiac catheterization data for Mr. A obtained from a combined right-and-left heart catheterization performed at rest*

Hemoglobin	136 g/L
Heart rate	76/min
O_2 consumption	255 ml O_2/min
O_2 capacity of arterial blood	190 ml O_2/L
Body surface area	1.81 m^2

Catheter site	Pressure (mm Hg)	O_2 Contents (ml O_2/L)
RA (Right atrium) (mean)	4	137
RV (Right ventricle) (sys./dias./end dias.)	27/2/10	137
PA (Pulmonary artery) (sys./dias./end dias.)	28/10/17	137
PCW (Pulmonary capillary wedge) (mean)	8	
LA (Left atrium) (mean)	8	181
LV (Left ventricle) (sys./dias./end dias.)	166/0/8	181
Ao (Aorta) (sys./dias./end dias.)	104/67/84	181

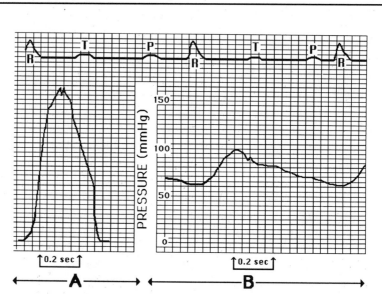

FIG. 7.1. Curves from Mr. A's catheterization. The upper curve is the EKG, and the lower curves represent LV pressure **(A)** and aortic pressure **(B)**. The pressure scale applies to both A and B.

ANSWERS TO QUESTIONS FOR PATIENT A

(1) **Tiredness** is rather nonspecific, but it's the kind of symptom that regularly brings people to seek medical advice. It often means that skeletal muscles aren't working properly. This could be related to intrinsic troubles with the muscles themselves (for example, muscular enzymatic dysfunctions) or to poor supply of either substrates or oxygen to the muscles. This in turn could be related to abnormalities in the associated systems, the pump, or the lung. On the other hand, all this machinery might well be intact, and the patient actually has a serious psychological depression. Invasive and expensive laboratory tests will often tell less about both the physical and mental status of any patient than a good history does.

Assuming practically but unrealistically that each of our problem patients is physiologically deranged, the tiredness reported to us should thus suggest heart, circulatory, or lung disease of at least 6 months duration. The possibilities at this point are legion, but the patient's age tends to rule out things like primary congenital heart defects; the time course (6 months) suggests that this is not a suddenly acquired pathological process; and the fact that Mr. A still plays golf means that he isn't deteriorating so rapidly that we can't take the time to do a proper history, conduct a physical, and obtain a set of laboratory tests before instituting therapy. We should also realize the possibility that Mr. A's occupation might somehow contribute to his symptomatology, although no major insights arise right now.

(2) **Palpitations,** sometime felt as a fluttering sensation in the chest or as an occasional extra strong heart beat, are usually indicative of an arrhythmia. This can range from isolated and unimportant premature atrial or ventricular beats to more serious tachycardias, which could reflect an underlying myocardial irritability secondary to a marginally adequate blood supply.

(3) **Shortness of breath** is usually a manifestation of increased respiratory drive. This could arise from processes that produce low

Pa_{O_2}, low arterial pH, or high Pa_{CO_2}. The causes of these are many, but the absence of this symptom makes it unlikely, for example, that Mr. A is suffering from pulmonary edema secondary to congestive heart failure. Inappropriate shortness of breath on exertion means that the lungs are not keeping the blood gases in line when cardiac output is increased.

(4) Sudden shortness of breath at night after retiring (paroxysmal nocturnal dyspnea) often means that a redistribution of blood to the pulmonary circuit has produced pulmonary (alveolar and perivascular) edema.

(5) Chest pain may reflect myocardial ischemia secondary to either pathological narrowing or spasm of the coronary arteries.

(6) Dizziness can come from an inadequate cerebral circulation, among other things, and this could have a cardiac origin.

(7) Ankle swelling usually indicates tissue edema secondary to extra high intracapillary pressures. This in turn could reflect right ventricular failure with the right ventricle's contractility so low that it cannot pump down the venous reservoir that feeds it. Other causes of edema should be thoroughly explored, however, if edema is found.

(8) A family history of heart disease should have made us suspicious that Mr. A was similarly afflicted. His lacking such a history does not rule out this possibility, however.

(9) An old physical exam often gives valuable blood pressure measurements and even usable diagnoses.

(10) A patient's general appearance is of paramount importance in evaluating just how sick he is and how long his disease may have been afflicting him. Prolonged congestive heart failure, for example, takes its toll on one's appearance.

(11) A regular pulse is important in relation to Mr. A's history of palpitations. Whereas chronic atrial fibrillation is now unlikely, episodic tachycardias are still a definite possibility.

(12) Both the systolic and diastolic **blood pressures** are on the low side but may nevertheless be normal for Mr. A. If they're indeed low, the cause could be myocardial, valvular, or circulatory in nature.

(13) The finding of **clear lungs** makes left heart failure or pneumonia less likely.

(14) The absence of peripheral **edema** on the other hand speaks against serious right heart failure.

(15) Hepatosplenomegaly frequently results from a backing up of blood in the great veins due to right heart failure.

(16) A prominent thrust at the location of the apical impulse indicates probable increased left ventricular activity.

(17) Detecting **cardiac enlargement** is not easy on a physical exam. A displaced apical impulse is probably more reliable, for example, than is an increased area of cardiac dullness determined by percussing (tapping) the chest.

(18) An ejection murmur of this magnitude is definitely abnormal. Its location seriously suggests turbulent blood flow through the aortic valve.

(19) Radiation of an ejection murmur to the neck implies even more strongly that there is trouble getting blood through the aortic valve.

(20) The loudest component of the **second heart sound** is usually caused by closure of the aortic valve. A soft second sound suggests further that the aortic valve is not well.

(21) Diagnostic possibilities after the history and physical:
The combination of tiredness, suggesting low relative cardiac output during exercise, a slightly low blood pressure at rest, and a systolic aortic valve murmur radiating into the neck point strongly to aortic valvular stenosis. So strong is the implication, that Mr. A was scheduled for an echocardiogram and cardiac catheterization to confirm the findings even before the results of routine lab tests appeared on the ward.

(22) These **blood tests** may be influenced by an acute myocardial infarction and associated destruction of muscle cells.

(23) Chest films reliably report large hearts, large pleural effusions, and significant pulmonary edema. They're not as reliable for determining left ventricular hypertrophy in the absence of cardiomegaly. (Hypertrophy here means an increase in muscle mass, whereas cardiomegaly means a larger heart. Note that the muscle mass could increase by encroaching on the ventricular cavity without increasing external ventricular size, and a heart can become larger by increasing its ventricular cavity without increasing muscle mass.)

(24) These **EKG** signs suggest left ventricular hypertrophy, but may give a significant number of false positives.

(25) Diagnostic possibilities after routine lab work: The chest film and EKG findings are consistent with left ventricular hypertrophy without cardiomegaly or frank heart failure. One would still worry at this point whether atherosclerotic heart disease was contributing to Mr. A's symptoms and might complicate an intended surgical repair of his aortic valve.

Cardiac Catheterization Results

(26) For **pulmonary blood flow,** use the Fick principle, dividing the O_2 consumption by the pulmonary arteriovenous O_2 content difference:

(ml O_2/min)/(ml O_2/L blood) = 255/(181 − 137) = 5.79 L/min

(27) For **pulmonary vascular resistance,** use Ohm's law, dividing the pressure gradient by the flow:

$$(17 − 8)/5.79 = 1.55 \text{ mm Hg}/(\text{L/min})$$

(28) For **systemic blood flow,** use the Fick principle again, this time with systemic O_2 contents:

$$255/(181 − 137) = 5.79 \text{ L/min}$$

(29) Cardiac index is obtained by dividing the cardiac output by the body surface area:

$$5.79/1.81 = 3.20 \text{ (L/min)}/\text{m}^2$$

(30) Systemic vascular resistance uses Ohm's law again, this time with systemic mean pressures:

$$(84 − 4)/5.79 = 13.8 \text{ mm Hg}/(\text{L/min})$$

(31) Left ventricular stroke volume is obtained by dividing the left ventricular output by the heart rate:

$$5{,}790/76 = 76 \text{ ml}$$

(32) There are no abnormal discontinuities in the pattern of O_2 **contents,** indicating that there is no abnormal shunting of blood. This helps to rule out congenital septal defects.

(33) There is a large systolic gradient in **pressures** between the LV and the aorta. This essentially clinches the diagnosis of aortic stenosis.

(34) The **cardiac index** is quite normal, showing that the heart has been able to keep the flow up in spite of the increased valvular resistance. This is often found in aortic valvular stenosis, with inadequate cardiac output first appearing during exercise, and only later at rest. When the cardiac index becomes low at rest, such patients often deteriorate rapidly. Mitral stenosis, on the other hand, may show a decreased cardiac index early in the development of the disease and be well tolerated because it is not a strain on the left ventricle.

(35) **Systemic vascular resistance** is on the low side, which is convenient considering the fact that the LV is already seeing a high resistance to its output through the aortic valve. Normal physiologic control mechanisms, on the other hand, might lead us to expect just the opposite: The low arterial pressure on the distal side of the aortic resistance would promote an increased arteriolar resistance via arterial baroreceptors. The explanation for the low systemic resistance found here is not immediately apparent.

(36) The aortic peak **pressure lags** the left ventricular peak:

R wave to LV peak = 0.16 sec, R wave to Ao peak = 0.28 sec
Lag = 0.28 − 0.16 = 0.12 sec

The lag, normally far smaller than this, can be attributed to the insertion of an aortic valvular resistance.

(37) This is merely your direct measurement of the reported **pressure gradient** in (33) above.

(38) The calculated **weighted mean pressure** is $(2 \times 67/3) + (104/3) = 79.3$ mm Hg. This is lower than the measured mean aortic pressure of 84 mm Hg because systolic pressure rise has been substantially blunted by the aortic valvular resistance.

(39) Figure 7.2 is a hypothetical **pressure/volume diagram** of Mr. A's left ventricle.

(40) Surgical replacement of this patient's stenotic aortic valve is clearly indicated and would probably be life saving.

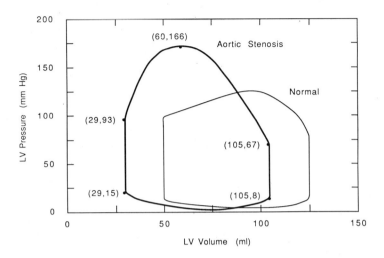

FIG. 7.2. **a:** Starting at the point where the mitral valve opens (end diastolic volume = 105 ml, end diastolic pressure = 8 mm Hg) and going counterclockwise consider the following features of Fig. 7.2. **b:** The first encountered phase of the cardiac cycle, isovolumetric contraction, is represented by a straight vertical line. **c:** The aortic valve opens at a pressure of 67 mm Hg, corresponding to diastolic pressure in the aorta. **d:** Thereafter, pressure continues to rise as volume falls, until a peak LV pressure of 166 mm Hg is achieved at some point between end diastolic and end systolic volume, here arbitrarily taken as 60 ml. **e:** Then pressure falls until the LV reaches end systolic volume, calculated as end diastolic volume minus stroke volume = 105 − 76 = 29 ml. The pressure at this point, 93 mm Hg, corresponds to aortic pressure at the dicrotic notch, which signals closing of the aortic valve. **f:** Pressure then falls on the vertical straight line in isovolumetric relaxation until a pressure of 15 mm Hg or so is reached. This pressure should be high enough so that the mean pressure during rapid and slow ventricular filling is somewhere near 8 mm Hg, the mean left atrial pressure. **g:** The lowest LV pressure, occurring near the end of rapid ventricular filling, should be 0 mm Hg.

PATIENT B

Chief Complaint

Mrs. B, a 35-year-old penny whistle player, was admitted to University Hospital complaining of mild chest pains in stressful situations for about 6 months **(1).**

Present Illness and Past History

Her pain was sharp but mild, and was felt over the left anterior chest. It did not radiate elsewhere and was not associated with exertion, eating, or exposure to cold (these pains suggest a musculoskeletal origin, rather than a cardiac one). Three months prior to admission a heart murmur was noted, and her right ventricle was found to be enlarged by echocardiography **(2)**.

There was no family history of heart disease.

Physical Exam

Mrs. B appeared to be a well-developed and nourished white female of her stated age in no obvious distress. Vital signs included a weight of 57 kg, temp. 37°C, pulse 85/min and regular, and blood pressure 102/66 mm Hg taken in the left arm sitting **(3)**. Her lungs were clear, and there was no edema or hepatosplenomegaly **(4)**. There was a right ventricular heave (sternal lift indicates a large, forceful right ventricle) **(5)** and a grade 2/6 systolic crescendo–decrescendo (ejection) murmur in the pulmonic area **(6)**. There was a fixed split of the second heart sound **(7)**.

Working Hypothesis

Think of some possible diagnostic categories and perhaps some specific diagnoses **(8)** and plan what tests you will administer **(9)**.

Laboratory

White count, differential, and LDH were all within normal limits (see Patient A). Chest films showed a slightly enlarged right ventricle and clear lung fields **(10)**. The EKG showed an incomplete right bundle branch block pattern **(11)**.

Working Hypothesis

Take a moment to assess your diagnostic choices thus far, and plan for more ambitious and expensive tests if you think they're really necessary (12).

Echocardiography

A two-dimensional echocardiograph showed the right ventricle (RV) to be enlarged without evident hypertrophy and the pulmonic valve leaflets to be mobile. Cold saline with dissolved air was injected intravenously, and the evolving small bubbles were seen to be deviated in the RA by a stream of blood issuing forth from the interatrial septum.

Cardiac Catheterization

Cardiac catheterization data are presented in Table 7.2. Are any of the O_2 contents or pressures abnormal (13)? How does this help you with the diagnosis (14)?

Using the data in Table 7.2, calculate the following, indicating appropriate units:

Pulmonary blood flow (15)
Systemic blood flow (16)
Cardiac index (17)
Right ventricular stroke volume (18)
Left ventricular stroke volume (19)
Pulmonary vascular resistance (20)
Systemic vascular resistance (21)

How has the body been able to accommodate the increased blood flow into the right atrium (22)?

Using the RV pressures and stroke volume obtained at cardiac catheterization and assuming an RV end-diastolic volume of 220 ml construct a pressure/volume diagram for the right ventricle (23).

What is your final diagnosis for Mrs. B (24)?

TABLE 7.2. *Cardiac catheterization data for Mrs. B*

Hemoglobin	134 g/L
Heart rate	85/min
O_2 consumption	219 ml O_2/min
O_2 capacity	186 ml O_2/L
Body surface area	1.52 m^2

Catheter site	Pressure (mm Hg)	O_2 Contents (ml O_2/L)
MV (Mixed venous)		131.4
RA (Right atrium) (mean)	8	163
RV (Right ventricle) (sys./dias./end dias.)	32/6/10	163
PA (Pulmonary artery) (sys./dias./mean)	30/15/22	163
PCW (Pulmonary capillary wedge) (mean)	9	
LA (Left atrium) (mean)	9	178
LV (Left ventricle) (sys./dias./end dias.)	106/5/12	178
Ao (Aorta) (sys./dias./mean)	102/66/84	178

ANSWERS TO QUESTIONS FOR PATIENT B

(1) Chest pain isn't as helpful as the tiredness of patient A. A young woman of this age is unlikely to have atherosclerotic heart disease, but we are obligated to do a thoughtful examination of the problem, if only to reassure the patient that we can find nothing wrong.

(2) With a more detailed history the chest pain seems even less likely to be due to coronary disease. However, it turns out that Mrs. B has recently been evaluated for heart disease, and does indeed have a **heart murmur** and **right ventricular enlargement** which will warrant further workup. The right ventricular enlargement can mean either an increased end diastolic volume (dilatation) or increased wall thickness (hypertrophy) or both.

(3) These **vital signs** are all within normal limits for a woman of this age.

(4) The absence of **fluid** in the lungs (which would cause them to make unusual sounds and not be clear) or fluid and blood accumulations in the systemic venous circulation suggests strongly that neither right nor left heart failure, respectively, is present.

(5) The **right ventricular heave** could mean either hypertrophy or dilatation.

(6) The placement of the **murmur** suggests that the pulmonic valve is affected, and the timing and quality of the murmur suggest that too much blood is being forced through a normal orifice or a normal flow is traversing a narrowed orifice.

(7) The second heart sound normally **splits** on inspiration and closes on expiration. The second component of the sound is due to closure of the pulmonic valve. When this component is persistently delayed, it may mean an increased flow of blood in the pulmonary circuit or a delayed activation (perhaps associated with a right His bundle branch block) of the right ventricle.

(8) In our **diagnostic possibilities** we should consider lesions capable of producing both a right ventricular hypertrophy (RVH) and an increased right ventricular flow. Left-to-right shunting via atrial or ventricular septal defects could be possible.

(9) We should **test** more thoroughly for RVH and possibly for shunting of blood. An EKG may show an RVH pattern, and both echocardiography and cardiac catheterization are probably indicated.

(10) **Clear lung fields** mean that left ventricular failure is unlikely.

(11) This **EKG pattern,** while found in a large percentage of the normal population, is found in most patients with an atrial septal defect (ASD).

(12) The **diagnostic possibilities** are already quite limited. The large right ventricle, fixed split second sound, pulmonic systolic murmur, and EKG findings strongly suggest an ASD, but because the definitive treatment of this is open heart surgery we should schedule Mrs. B for echocardiography and cardiac catheterization to confirm our impression. An occult pulmonic valve stenosis (narrowing), for example, would require an entirely different operation.

(13) The O_2 **content** rises (131.4 to 163) instead of remaining constant as blood flows from the calculated mixed venous compartment to the right atrium (RA) in this patient. The O_2 contents from left atrium (LA) through Ao are all lower than the approximate 200 value we have considered before in the text. Catheterization **pressures** all seem within normal limits.

(14) The increase in O_2 content in the RA probably results from an admixture of highly oxygenated blood from the left atrium (LA) entering the RA via an atrial septal defect. Low arterial O_2 contents reflect the somewhat low O_2 capacity (186), which in turn is a manifestation of a slightly low hemoglobin. The calculated arterial saturation (178/186 = 0.96 or 96%) is perfectly normal.

(15) For **pulmonary blood flow** use the Fick principle, dividing the O_2 consumption by the pulmonary arteriovenous O_2 content difference:

$$(ml\ O_2/min)/(ml\ O_2/L\ blood) = 219/(178 - 163) = 14.6\ L/min$$

Note that this value is roughly three times a normal resting cardiac output, meaning that the lungs are being perfused at a comparably elevated level.

(16) For **systemic blood flow** use the Fick principle again, this time with systemic O_2 contents:

$$219/(178 - 131.4) = 4.70\ L/min$$

This value is a normal resting cardiac output, existing at the same time as the elevated pulmonary flow calculated above. The explanation is a shunt of $14.6 - 4.7 = 9.9$ L/min from LA to RA through the atrial septal defect.

(17) Cardiac index is obtained by dividing the systemic cardiac output by the body surface area:

$$4.70/1.52 = 3.09 \ (L/min)/m^2$$

(18) Right ventricular stroke volume is obtained by dividing the right ventricular output by the heart rate:

$$14{,}600/85 = 172 \ ml$$

(19) Left ventricular stroke volume is obtained by dividing the left ventricular output by the heart rate:

$$4{,}700/85 = 55 \ ml$$

indicating the LV has less work to do.

(20) For **pulmonary vascular resistance** use Ohm's law, dividing the mean pressure gradient by the flow:

$$(22 - 9)/14.9 = 0.87 \ mm \ Hg/(L/min)$$

(21) Systemic vascular resistance uses Ohm's law again, this time with systemic mean pressures:

$$(84 - 8)/4.70 = 16 \ mm \ Hg/(L/min)$$

(22) The body seems to have accommodated the increased right atrial input flow by pumping it through the lungs. This requires somewhat higher than normal right ventricular pressures. Later in the course of this disease (ASD) many patients develop a fixed higher-than-normal pulmonary vascular resistance, which eventually may result in right ventricular failure. The mechanism for the formation of this increased resistance is unknown.

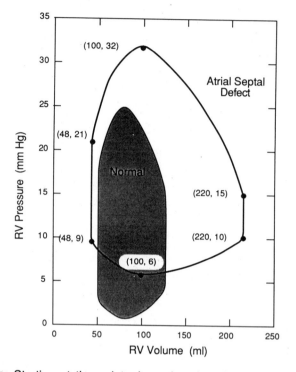

FIG. 7.3. **a:** Starting at the point where the tricuspid valve closes (end diastolic volume = 220 ml, end diastolic pressure = 10 mm Hg) and going counter-clockwise, consider the following features of Fig. 7.3. **b:** The first encountered phase of the cardiac cycle, isovolumetric contraction, is represented by a straight vertical line. **c:** The pulmonic valve opens at a pressure of 15 mm Hg, corresponding to diastolic pressure in the pulmonary artery. **d:** Thereafter, pressure continues to rise as volume falls, until a peak RV pressure of 32 mm Hg is achieved at some point between end diastolic and end systolic volume, here arbitrarily taken as 100 ml. **e:** Then pressure falls until the RV reaches end systolic volume, calculated as end diastolic volume minus stroke volume = 220 − 172 = 48 ml. The pressure at this point, 21 mm Hg (arbitrarily taken), corresponds to the closing of the pulmonic valve. **f:** Pressure then falls on the vertical straight line in isovolumetric relaxation until a pressure of 9 mm Hg or so is reached. This pressure should be high enough so that the mean pressure during rapid and slow ventricular filling is somewhere near 8 mm Hg, the mean right atrial pressure. **g:** The lowest RV pressure, occurring near the end of rapid ventricular filling, should be 6 mm Hg, the lowest pressure in the ventricular cycle.

(23) See Fig. 7.3 for pressure/volume diagram of Mrs. B's right ventricle.

(24) As suspected even prior to echocardiography and cardiac catheterization, Mrs. B's **diagnosis** should be interatrial septal defect with left to right shunt.

PATIENT C

Chief Complaint

Mr. C, a 47-year-old salesman, was admitted to University Hospital complaining of severe chest pain of 1-hr duration **(1)**.

Present Illness

Mr. C's pain was sudden in onset, while moving furniture, and was said to be "heavy" and "pressing" over his sternum with radiation to his jaw **(2)**. It was accompanied by feelings of nausea and shortness of breath **(3)**, with the latter persisting to the time of admission.

Past History

There was no previous history of chest pain or heart trouble, except that Mr. C's father had died of a heart attack at age 50 **(4)**. Review of his other systems was noncontributory.

Physical Exam

Mr. C appeared to be a white male of about his stated age in acute distress from chest pain and shortness of breath. He was somewhat disoriented, not knowing the day of the week or the city, and his skin was cold and clammy **(5)**. His pulse was 130/min **(6)** and irregular, with frequent premature beats being associated with compensatory pauses **(7)**. Blood pressure was 90/50 mm Hg in the left arm, taken in the supine position **(8)**. Heart sounds were soft, and no murmurs were heard **(9)**. The lungs disclosed crackling inspiratory râles at both bases, but no areas of dullness **(10)**. There was no hepatosplenomegaly **(11)**.

Working Hypothesis

Make an assessment and plan your further tests and therapy, remembering that some aspects of a cardiac catheterization may be performed at the bedside using a flow-directed venous catheter **(12)**.

Laboratory

An EKG was taken. Predict the results before turning to the report **(13)**. A chest film was taken. Again, predict the results **(14)**.

Hospital Course

An intravenous, flow-directed, Swann Gans catheter was placed, allowing the measurement of a critical physiological variable. What was it **(15)**? The right ventricular systolic pressure, also measured using this catheter, was 50 mm Hg. Why **(16)**?

Treatment was instituted with intravenous pronestyl, lidocaine (also having local anesthetic action), and inderal (a beta-adrenergic blocker) to decrease myocardial irritability and lessen the chance of ventricular tachycardia arising. What would be a common important side effect of these drugs in Mr. C **(17)**?

Cardiac output was measured at 2.0 L/min, using a bedside thermodilution method. Knowing that heart rate is 140 beats/min and body surface area is 1.72 m^2, calculate the cardiac index **(18)** and stroke volume **(19)**.

A wedge pressure of 22 mm Hg (see answer to question 15) reflects a serious load on the heart. What is the nature of this load, and how should it be treated **(20)?**

Mr. C responded well to the therapy in that his cardiac output rose to 3.5 L/min with essentially no change in blood pressure. His mental status improved. Digitalis proved ineffective in further increasing cardiac output. Using a plot of both venous return and cardiac output versus left atrial pressure, trace Mr. C's status from (a) his normal state (b) his acute myocardial infarction to (c) his immediate physiological response and to (d) his response to therapy in the hospital **(21).**

He was later discharged on sublingual vasodilator therapy, and was able to resume his normal activities within 8 months. His final diagnosis was cardiogenic shock secondary to an acute myocardial infarction.

ANSWERS TO QUESTIONS FOR PATIENT C

(1) It's best to deal with an **acute chest pain** as a potential myocardial infarction (possible coronary occlusion) until proven otherwise.

(2) These **characteristics of the pain** brand it as coronary artery disease, and strongly suggest an ongoing infarct.

(3) The **shortness of breath** probably means that blood is backing up in the pulmonary circulation, producing pulmonary edema. This process is most likely due to acute left ventricular failure, with the left ventricle unable to pump down the reservoir of blood feeding it.

(4) Coronary artery disease runs in families. This finding makes a congenital malformation less likely as a cause of Mr. C's symptoms.

(5) Disorientation results in this case from poor cerebral perfusion, secondary to pump failure. **Cold, clammy skin** results from the same cause with superimposed vasoconstriction making skin blood flow even lower. Decreased or absent urine flow will result from similar mechanisms.

(6) Elevated pulse rate can be a reflex response to a low blood pressure via arterial baroreceptors.

(7) A poorly perfused myocardium is irritable, and this is often manifested by the acute onset of **premature ventricular beats.** The compensatory pause found here makes this diagnosis even more likely.

(8) The **low blood pressure** should come as no surprise because we've already seen some of its consequences. The problem is one of lowered overall myocardial contractility, with some of the cardiac muscle either weak or not functional.

(9) The **soft heart sounds** may reflect low contractility.

(10) The **basilar râles** reflect an abnormal accumulation of alveolar fluid, that is, pulmonary edema secondary to left ventricular failure.

(11) Hepatosplenomegaly would reflect high systemic venous pressure secondary to right ventricular failure. This apparently has not occurred here.

(12) This looks like a clear-cut case of an acute myocardial infarction with shock resulting from the extremely low contractility remaining. We should check more directly for lung fluid and heart size by getting a chest film, and we should confirm our suspicions about his premature beats and the presence of an evolving infarction by getting an EKG.

The medical problem is to somehow unload the heart so that healing and recovery can take place. Myocardial wall stress during systole represents this load and depends directly on both ventricular volume (radius) and developed transmural (approximately aortic) pressure, as is seen from the law of Laplace: $S = Pr/(2h)$, in which S is stress in pressure units, P is the transmural pressure, r is the effective chamber radius, and h is wall thickness. P is already as low as can readily sustain life, so we must try to find out whether the left ventricle is large and dilated. Signs and symptoms already point to a high pulmonary venous–left atrial pressure which would be directly related to end diastolic ventricular size, so we should measure and monitor this variable if possible. Wedging a venous catheter transiently in the pulmonary bed will give us just such an estimate of pulmonary venous pressure.

(13) The **EKG** showed frequent premature ventricular complexes in a bigeminal pattern. (This is indicative of myocardial irritability.) There was also elevation of the ST segment in the anterolateral chest leads, consistent with an acute myocardial infarction.

(14) The **chest film** showed increased bronchial markings and fluid at both lung bases, consistent with mild pulmonary edema. There was biventricular enlargement.

(15) The **critical variable** is the left atrial pressure, measured indirectly here as the pulmonary capillary wedge pressure. The value was 22 mm Hg, to be compared with normal values of approximately 5–12 mm Hg. It indicates a high pressure in the pulmonary veins and hence in the left ventricle at end diastole. It reflects severe left ventricular failure and indicates a large ventricular size.

(16) The **right ventricular pressure** was elevated in order to push blood through the lungs against the large back pressure in the pulmonary veins. This is a normal compensation, but also a load on the right ventricle.

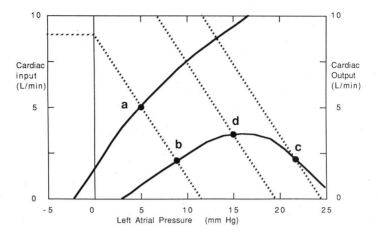

FIG. 7.4. Prior to his infarct Mr. C was probably operating near point **a** above. With coronary occlusion, he suffered an abrupt decrease in contractility, moving from his normal isocontractility line (*dark line*) down along his original venous filling line (*dashed line*) to point **b.** Very soon thereafter his baroreceptor system sensed the very low blood pressure accompanying this extremely low cardiac output and activated the sympathetics to increase venous tone. This moved Mr. C's operating point along the "bad" isocontractility line from **b** to **c,** thus increasing cardiac output somewhat over the situation at **b.** This latter movement is an example of the Starling effect. It represents an overcorrection in terms of venous tone in that the ventricle is so stretched that it is working at too great a wall stress, and cardiac output actually falls with increasing stretch. Vasodilator therapy undoes some of this Starling effect, moving the operating point back to **d** where operation is more efficient at a lower wall stress.

  A caveat: This type of diagram greatly oversimplifies the situation. Heart rate changes are not reflected and venous resistance is not changed (parallel venous tone curves). Not all investigators would agree with the falling off of cardiac output on the lower isocontractility curve, although the clinical phenomena remain: Vasodilator therapy improves volume-overloaded patients in heart failure.

(17) Anesthetics and beta-blockers both decrease myocardial contractility. Using them here gambles that their therapeutic effects will outweigh their further depression of contractility.

(18) Cardiac index is cardiac output divided by body surface area:

$$2.0/1.72 = 1.16 \ (L/min)/m^2$$

a very low value, indicative of LV failure in Mr. C.

(19) Stroke volume is cardiac output divided by heart rate:

$$2,000/140 = 14 \ ml$$

less than 3 teaspoonfuls per beat.

(20) The **load on the heart** has to do with wall stress (see answer to question 12). Because the pressure should not be lowered further the only variable to attack is ventricular radius (or volume). Vasodilating the patient will give his circulating blood volume more room to flow into and will thus decompress all circulatory compartments, including the left atrium and ventricle. Accordingly, a nitroprusside drip was instituted.

(21) See Fig. 7.4, the input/output (Guyton) diagram of the course of Mr. C's illness.

Subject Index